TRAINING + COMPETING WITH A
CONTINUOUS GLUCOSE MONITOR

TRAINING + COMPETING WITH A
CONTINUOUS GLUCOSE MONITOR

A USER'S GUIDE FOR ATHLETES

Hunter Allen

Text copyright © 2025 Hunter Allen. Design and concept copyright © 2025 VeloPress. All rights reserved. Any unauthorized duplication in whole or in part or dissemination of this edition by any means (including but not limited to photocopying, electronic devices, digital versions, and the internet) will be prosecuted to the fullest extent of the law.

CrossFit® is a registered trademark of CrossFit, LLC.
Ironman® is a registered trademark of World Triathlon Corporation.

Published by:

an imprint of Ulysses Press
32 Court Street, Suite 2109
Brooklyn, NY 11201
www.velopress.com

VeloPress is the leading publisher of books on sports for passionate and dedicated athletes around the world. Focused on cycling, triathlon, running, swimming, nutrition/diet, and more, VeloPress books help you achieve your goals and reach the top of your game.

ISBN: 978-1-64604-693-5
Library of Congress Control Number: 2024931675

Printed in Canada
10 9 8 7 6 5 4 3 2 1

Project editor: Kierra Sondereker
Managing editor: Claire Chun
Front cover design: Rebecca Lown
Design and layout: Westchester Publishing Services

Figure 4.1 (p. 51) courtesy of Jeffrey Rothschild. Table 7.0 (p. 121) courtesy of Dr. Michael Riddell.

Please note: This book has been written and published strictly for informational purposes, and in no way should be used as a substitute for consultation with health care professionals. You should not consider educational material herein to be the practice of medicine or to replace consultation with a physician or other medical practitioner. The author and publisher are providing you with information in this work so that you can have the knowledge and can choose, at your own risk, to act on that knowledge. The author and publisher also urge all readers to be aware of their health status and to consult health care professionals before beginning any health program.

This book is independently authored and published and no sponsorship or endorsement of this book by, and no affiliation with, any celebrities, products, brands, or other copyright and trademark holders mentioned within is claimed or suggested. All trademarks that appear in this book belong to their respective owners and are used here for informational purposes only. The author and publisher encourage readers to patronize the brands mentioned in this book.

Contents

Introduction vii
Preface: An Introduction to CGMs xi

1	What Is a CGM?	1
2	How Foods Impact Your Glucose and Performance	17
3	The Steps to Using Your CGM	33
4	Using a CGM for Optimal Training, Competing, and Recovery	49
5	Strategies on CGM Use for Performance	75
6	Learn From Others' Data	93
7	Diabetes and Athletic Performance: Using a CGM	111
8	Using Your CGM for Longevity and Vitality	129
9	Putting It All Together	149

Appendix A 153
Notes 157
Glossary 169
Index 173
Acknowledgments 179
About the Author 181

Introduction

THIS BOOK IS FOR PEOPLE WHO ARE INTERESTED in optimizing their blood sugar levels for performance. This book is not for people who want to know exactly which carbohydrate, drink, or gel they should take before, during, or after exercise. There are tremendously well-written and researched books that explain exactly the perfect ratios of glucose and fructose, and the right nutrition one should have to improve hydration and for prolonged performance. This book will help you to understand how to keep your blood glucose levels stable, how to raise them when you need to, when to recognize that your glucose levels are low, and how and when you should address this. A continuous glucose monitor (CGM) can improve athletic performance in training and when competing. When you achieve a great understanding of how to recognize the different scenarios that your blood glucose goes through not only during your day, but also when exercising and training, you'll be able to optimize your blood glucose for peak performance.

This book is *not* for type 1 and type 2 diabetics that are looking for answers on how to better control their insulin levels or reverse their type 2 diabetes. There are many other good books about those subjects. While I do have a chapter that discusses how type 1 and type 2 diabetics can better use a CGM for performance, it's just that—for performance. So if you're a type 1 or type 2 diabetic, you *will* find very useful information here. I encourage you to read the entire book thoroughly, as you'll find "nuggets" throughout that will help you improve your athletic performance.

In spending over two years researching, learning, questioning, and traveling the world finding out about so many topics related to blood glucose carbohydrate, absorption performance, and endocrinology insulin, I've been able to figure out patterns and correlations, and have come up with some helpful ways to optimize all these things so that you can improve your performance. Many of these things are correlations, and it's important that you don't take correlations as conclusions or causation. A correlation is when two variables are linearly related. For example, you might see your glucose level jump to 200 milligrams per deciliter (mg/dL) every time you eat a doughnut and think these are correlated, but you might not consider that you had three tablespoons of sugar in your coffee 15 minutes before that doughnut. So, while it appears that eating a doughnut is the cause of the glucose spike and the two are correlated, you're missing an important factor that needs to be taken into account for true causation. It generally is highly useful and very interesting when you see different correlations, but it's also important to do the testing yourself so that you can discover what works for you and what doesn't.

The next thing to keep in mind is that there are many variables that will impact your blood glucose response. Some of these variables are: gender; age; fitness level; length of your workouts; intensity of your workouts; training freshness or fatigue; amount and quality of sleep; regular alcohol usage (including the night before); your gut microbiome; which macro diet you are on, like vegan or paleo, etc.; your prediabetic symptoms; and more. Not only do these variables play a role, but you can also change your responses based on your changes in health, such as weight loss and improvements in eating. So you could have a particular response at the beginning of this journey, but through increased fitness, weight loss, improved eating habits, a change in diet, and better sleep, you might need to completely re-read this book a year from now to understand the "new" you. This is just one reason why learning how to use your CGM for performance can be challenging. On a smaller scale, you might find that "X" food gives you a "Y" response on Monday, but on Friday, "X" food gives you a "Z" response. It's *imperative* that you keep this in mind as you watch your blood glucose values, train, eat, and read this book.

This book is also the culmination of an important journey to improve my own longevity, vitality, and performance having battled hypoglycemia many times when racing as an amateur and professional cyclist. Unfortunately, I have a family history of cardiovascular disease, high cholesterol, high blood pressure, type 2 diabetes, and stroke. My mother had type 2 diabetes and at age 58 had a quintuple bypass. She died of a stroke at age 63. My father had a quintuple bypass at 55 years old, has had two stents since then at age 76, and has battled throughout his life with high blood pressure. My grandmother on my mom's side died of a massive heart attack at age 63. My grandfather, on my father's side and whom I never met, also died of a massive heart attack at age 44. So the odds are against me! I have had borderline poor lipid scores all my life:

- Triglycerides/high-density lipoprotein (TG/HDL) ratio = 2.73 (ratio of 2 or less is excellent);
- Apolipoprotein B (ApoB) = 100 mg/dL (less than 90 mg/dL is ideal); and
- Lipoprotein(a) (Lp(a)) = 109 nanomoles per liter (nmol/L) (less than 75 is ideal).

My hemoglobin (HbA1c) has hovered between 5.7 and 6.3 for nearly 20 years now. I have had my blood work tested almost every six months for over 30 years, along with multiple stress tests, calcium scans, and even a CT angiogram. So far, everything has been perfect with my heart—no blockages of any sort. I attribute this to being a lifelong endurance cyclist and someone that does strenuous cardiovascular exercise nearly every day. However, I also know that diet has played a role in this and, while I have done my best over the years, I know I could do better. I have recently changed my diet, which has improved my numbers (more about that in Chapter 8, which is on longevity and vitality). After having spent over two and a half years researching for this book, learning about my blood glucose and the glucose responses of the athletes that I coach and work with, and reading hundreds of scientific studies, I believe that maintaining a lower and more stable blood glucose level is one of the most important things I can do for my cardiovascular health. Using a CGM has made a profound difference in my average daily and nightly blood glucose levels, has held me accountable to the choices I make in my diet, and I believe it has been a significant contributor to improving my longevity and vitality.

One of the hardest parts about writing this book was the organization of the material. There are many concepts, ideas, responses, etc. that easily could fit in multiple chapters. This means that for you, the reader, it's important that you read the whole book. You might skip around in chapters but be sure that you read the entire book. There might be a performance enhancing concept that is explained in Chapter 4, which also has a longevity and vitality impact you should know about in Chapter 8. As you read this, I hope you find yourself looking at the graphs and charts and saying to yourself, "I have seen that before in my data. Now I know what it means." That's been a key goal of mine in writing this book: to help you understand the responses, learn why something is or isn't happening and then decide which "arrow in the quiver" you want to shoot next for that situation. You will also find yourself saying, "But, what about when this happens or that happens?" I ask you to be patient and read the entire book as it's likely your scenario will be explained in a later chapter. Possibly, it's not explained at all and that's also been a challenge in writing this book. If I covered every glucose response this book would be 1,000 pages long and not very interesting for most readers. As we all continue to learn more about using a CGM for performance, I'll put new insights and ideas into my website: www.TrainingandCompetingwithaCGM.com. Please feel free to reach out to me and my team when you've learned a new insight or have seen a new response and don't know what it means or what to do about it.

Full disclosure: I am not a scientist, nor do I play one on the internet. I am a very keen and knowledgeable cycling coach that happens to have spent the last 25 years working with bicycle power meters and analyzing power data. I also co-founded the TrainingPeaks software, so I intimately know the ins and outs of data analysis. I am very good at statistics, understanding patterns, trends, and correlations. This book is not a gold standard double-blinded placebo-controlled trial of athletes' blood glucose values. They all knew they had a CGM, saw their numbers and were influenced (or not!) by them throughout the examples, charts, and graphs that you'll read about. At the same time, the data that you'll see is the data. It's not like anyone was able to fake their blood glucose values or change them after the fact. I hope as you read this book, you'll find that I have created a well-balanced book that blends in science where it's needed (with high-quality references backing up those statements), an approachable reading style so that everyone can understand and apply the principles, and nuggets of information throughout so that you can improve your performance. This book is not attempting to appear in any scientific journals. I offer it to you so that you can use what I and others have learned to make your own decisions and act when needed. I also hope it helps to improve your longevity and vitality.

....

It's very important to remember that this book does not replace your doctor,
and is not offering medical advice in any way. It's important that you
consult your physician when making any changes to your health that
could change your prescription medication and/or change
your blood glucose values.

....

Preface: An Introduction to CGMs

ALL OVER THE WORLD PEOPLE ARE MEASURING their glucose levels to better understand how to stay healthy, how to improve performance, and how to make positive behavioral changes. Continuous glucose monitors (CGMs) have been in use since the early 2000s, but their accuracy was so good that in 2016, the US Food and Drug Administration (FDA) approved CGM readings to replace fingerstick measuring. People with type 1 and type 2 diabetes have been using CGMs since that time to better understand how much insulin to use, what the impact of foods are on their glucose, and how to change their diet to control their glucose levels throughout the day and night. It's only been since 2022, when the 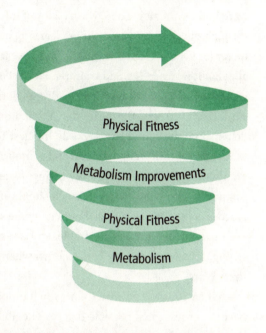 company Supersapiens launched Abbott's Libre Sense Glucose Sport Biosensor, that athletes have had access to CGMs and their glucose data. Up to that point, scientists, researchers, and doctors around the world really didn't know what non-diabetes users' glucose levels might be, how they reacted to certain foods, and what happened to their glucose levels during exercise, sleep and throughout all aspects of life. Scientists, researchers, and doctors only knew about glucose responses from their studies on people with type 1 and 2 diabetes. So it has been with some shock, surprise, and excitement that they're learning the responses in people without diabetes, including athletes.

Whether you're a bodybuilder, cyclist, CrossFitter, pickleball player or simply an active person that wants to stay healthy, you can improve your performance by learning about, understanding, and making changes to your behavior just by using a CGM to track your glucose levels. Whether you're a recreational athlete just looking to improve your health with more effective workouts at the gym, or you're a professional triathlete looking to win your next full-distance triathlon, a CGM can help you. It's an incredibly exciting and effective wearable that gives the user more insight into their body on a continuous basis, allowing them to make better fueling decisions in training, competition, and in daily life. Aaron Stevenson, a motorcycle coach and masters age cyclist, said this when he started using a CGM:

"For over 50 years, I have been riding and racing bicycles and motorcycles, and coaching professionally for the last 25 years. In the 1970s, sport nutrition, biometrics and training data were in their infancy. There wasn't a lot of information available for young athletes. I came up through the heart rate monitor era learning how to use heart rate zones, then bought a power meter for my bicycle and learned how to use it. Now, this biometric data allows me to personally monitor my eating and training habits. I'm seeing just how important it is to understand what my blood glucose levels are during all of my exercise. When I teach a weekend motorcycle clinic, I am full blast the entire day. While I don't show it to my athletes, internally, I'm really depleted by the end of the day. I do my best to eat snacks throughout the day, but now I see that I am not eating enough food and sometimes eat the wrong foods. Using the CGM uncovered some misconceptions in my eating. As an athlete, I want to properly fuel my body, and unknowingly, I consumed too much simple sugar like bananas and granola bars that had my glucose on a roller coaster all day. With some small but significant changes, I have been able to keep my glucose levels more stable, so I am still kicking it at the end of the day and feeling strong. It truly opened my eyes to learn what I have 'unknowingly' been doing to my body all these years!"[1]

When you start using a CGM, you'll unlock information about your body that you could have never imagined possible before. The ability to learn how your glucose fluctuates on an hourly, daily, and monthly basis, can inspire you to take action each day to improve your workouts, your recovery, and your competitions. Not only will a CGM help you with your performances, but it will also help you to improve your glucose stability in your daily life so that your energy levels are more stable, you have a better mood, and you reduce both the inflammation in your body and the high glucose values that could be doing damage to your body.

All the new numbers and data points coming out of commercial use CGMs aren't very useful for making behavioral changes if you don't understand them, contextualize them, or recognize the patterns in them. A clear step-by-step method to turn your CGM into a true tool and improve performance is the key to creating a great habit loop. Chapter 1 will teach the basics about CGMs, glucose, insulin, and the factors that influence your glucose readings. Chapter 2 will give you critical information in helping you to learn more about your individual response to foods, including some useful tips about eating foods in the correct order. Chapter 3 will lead you on the steps to becoming a pro user of a CGM. Learning about and understanding exactly what all the "squiggly" lines and numbers mean is critical to taking action and making changes, if needed, and that's why Chapters 4 and 5 are dedicated to teaching you to read CGM data in an easy-to-understand manner. Chapter 6 will dig into the science around CGMs, managing your glucose levels, and improving athletic performance. Chapter 7 will focus on how best to use a CGM and improve performance if you're an athlete with type 1 or type 2 diabetes. Chapter 8 will be the most popular chapter, as you'll learn about how to increase your longevity, vitality, and overall health. Your new wearable is going to be more than just an interesting number: it's going to help you to make decisions at every meal, every workout and every competition. It truly will become, for you, an optimal performance tool.

WHY SHOULD YOU USE A CGM AND CARE ABOUT YOUR GLUCOSE?

Before we dive into the specifics on what exactly a CGM is and how to use it, let's look at all the benefits that can come from reading this book and learning about monitoring your glucose levels.

Improved Athletic Performance

If your glucose levels are low or they drop below a certain threshold during exercise, then you'll be unable to perform at your best or possibly at all. Low blood sugar (glucose), or hypoglycemia, makes training and/or competing nearly impossible. Hypoglycemia, or "bonking" as cyclists call it, or "hitting the wall" as runners call it, usually occurs when your glucose level falls below 70 milligrams per deciliter (mg/dL). This can give you shakiness, dizziness, headache, muscle weakness, confusion, and, of course, hunger. Your body continually optimizes to maintain your glucose levels in a narrow range, which is called homeostasis. When you exercise, your liver releases stored glucose (called glycogen) into your bloodstream so your cells can make energy. At the same time, you ingest additional carbohydrates from food, which replaces the glucose used during exercise and helps to maintain glucose levels so that you can use these easily, and preserve stored glycogen. These two combinations allow you to perform at a high level of intensity and for a much longer time.

If your glucose is constantly dropping and you're not ingesting more carbohydrates, there will be only so long that you can exercise. Your muscles contain enough glycogen for 60 to 120 minutes of intense exercise, and your liver contains between 30 minutes of stored glycogen for a total combined possible amount of 2.5 hours of stored glycogen. For optimal performance in events longer than two hours, you'll want to eat carbohydrates before these glycogen supplies are depleted. By eating the correct type of carbohydrates at the right time, you can carefully regulate your glucose to maintain an optimal level before, during, and after your workouts and/or competitions. Ensuring you're fueling correctly before your events allows you to start your competitions ready to compete from the time the gun goes off. Recognizing during your exercise the different scenarios that your glucose levels might undergo, will keep you informed so that you can decide whether you need to ingest a quick acting carbohydrate or a slower acting carbohydrate. What you eat after your workout is just as important, especially if you're planning on working out the next day. Your CGM will help you track your recovery. It will give you insights on optimal foods to consume after the workout or before bedtime in order to improve recovery.

Establish Your Baseline Glucose and Your Glucose Performance Zone

For the first two weeks after applying your CGM your focus is on gathering and observing the data. Resist the temptation to change your diet. Make sure to make "ranges" around your meals (including before, during, and after eating until your glucose comes back down again), exercise, sleep, and stressful situations. This will allow you to see your peak glucose value, how fast it gets to its maximum (time-to-response), your average for that specific time, and how long it takes for your glucose to come back down. This will also allow you to establish your baseline (basal) glucose value. What is your norm? Generally, during the day, does your glucose hang around 90 mg/dL? 100 mg/dL? This could be considered your daily "pre-meal or pre-exercise" baseline. Theoretically, your true "baseline" is measured only in the morning after an overnight fast. Both of these, your daily baseline and your true morning baseline, could change over the course of the next six months, so write it down in the margin of this book with a date beside it.

Optimizing your glucose for workouts and competitions is an important way to ensure that you're performing at the highest level of your current fitness. It's not a guarantee of success by any means. That comes down to your training, strategy, coaching, desire to win, etc. However, what it can do, is ensure that you'll have plenty of energy for your event by keeping it in the right zone. You'll learn more about your glucose performance zone (GPZ) and how to find it in Chapter 3.

More Stable Energy Throughout Your Workout and Day

When your blood glucose levels drop, you begin to feel lethargic, sleepy, and you might even find yourself in a bad mood. And, of course, you won't be as productive as when your glucose is higher versus when it's close to your baseline, and stable. When you're on a roller coaster of high glucose then low glucose, it's hard to perform well throughout your workout, and it's tough on your liver, pancreas, and even your brain as you try to focus and concentrate. High blood glucose is not as big of a problem if you're staying below 200 mg/dL, which is around the top limit for normal healthy athletes that don't have type 1 or 2 diabetes. However, high glucose is not something you're striving for. More is not better in this case, as high blood glucose levels can cause inflammation, damage to the internal walls of your arteries and vessels, and puts a large strain on your pancreas to secrete more and more insulin to stabilize your body back to its basal level.[2]

A stable glucose, and it doesn't have to be perfect, will allow you to perform at a high level, be focused throughout your workout and/or competition, and will ultimately help you to focus on what's important, whether that's the next point in your tennis game, the next hill on your bicycle, or the next set of weights at the gym.

Be Accountable to Your Diet

Like any measuring tool, whether that is a heart rate monitor, stopwatch, or step counter, once you become aware of something and you can measure that thing, you'll improve it. Take that measuring tool away and you lose the ability to know what exactly is happening and, in this case, what is happening inside your body and how it reacts to ingested foods. I know that when I am using my CGM, I still make different food choices even after having used one now for over two years. I know that eating tortilla chips will absolutely blow up my blood glucose to over 200 mg/dL every time I have some, but if I don't have a CGM on, I'll reach for that bag of chips! Even athletes that I coach have said to me, "Woohoo, I am off sensor! I'll have that big pastry please," when we have stopped during a training ride out cycling. The accountability factor of using a CGM is a real thing, and it can keep you on track.

Improve Your Metabolic Health

What is metabolic health? Great question! There is no universally agreed-upon definition of metabolic health, but some scientists and doctors define it as the absence of metabolic concerns. Low abdominal fat, low triglycerides (less than 150 mg/dL), low-fasting blood glucose (less than 100 mg/dL), low blood pressure (less than 130/85 millimeters of mercury (mmHg)), and low high-density lipoprotein cholesterol (40 mg/dL or less in men and 50 mg/dL or less in women) are all indicators of good metabolic health.[3] Improving your metabolism, which is the conversion of foods to energy in your body, can directly impact your ability to perform at any level in athletics. If you can more efficiently convert foods into the substrates your body needs to perform well, then you'll be able to perform at an increasingly higher level in your chosen sport. The great news is that all the training you currently do *also* improves your metabolic health, including making you more sensitive to insulin, reducing the risks of disease, type 2 diabetes, and nonalcoholic fatty liver disease. At the same time, training also helps to improve your numbers in the five indicators of good metabolic health (mentioned at the start of this paragraph). So, it's an upward spiral of improvement. Exercise more, improve your metabolism and metabolic health, wear a CGM, understand how your glucose level responds, and make better choices to further improve your glucose stability and therefore metabolic health.

Reduce Your Risk of Type 2 Diabetes

Yes, athletes can get type 2 diabetes! In the book, *The Great Cholesterol Myth*, authors Dr. Jonny Bowden and Dr. Stephen Sinatra wrote, "Insulin resistance is the root cause of heart disease and insulin resistance is essentially an error of metabolism."[4] Dr. Robert Lustig, the author of *Metabolical*, said, "Emerging evidence shows that insulin resistance is the most important predictor of cardiovascular disease and type 2 diabetes."[5]

Type 2 diabetes, or adult-onset diabetes, occurs when your cells become resistant to insulin. Cells need insulin to "open the door" for glucose to go into the cell, but in type 2 diabetes, these cells no longer respond to insulin and therefore leave the glucose molecules to circulate in the bloodstream. A type 2 diabetic could have a glucose value as high as 400 mg/dL, whereas anything over 140 mg/dL is considered inflammatory to the body and causes damage to the epithelial (inner) layer of the vessels and arteries. This damage is then fixed by plaque and eventually the plaque becomes thick and hardened, and finally so clogged that blood flow is stopped, which results in a stroke or heart attack. Let's prevent that! And yes, even athletes can have clogged arteries. There are countless stories of well-known and little-known lifelong endurance athletes that have had heart attacks because of clogged arteries. Diet also plays a *huge* role as well, and you can't out-exercise a bad diet. Repeat after me: "You can't out-exercise a bad diet."[6]

Measuring your glucose value on a minute-by-minute basis throughout the day with a CGM makes you acutely aware of every increase or decrease in your glucose, which in turn helps you to correlate the foods that you eat with your glucose response and then make better decisions for your health and sport. When you create more stability and less variability in your average daily glucose, you'll undoubtedly improve your insulin sensitivity. Couple this with a healthy diet that is high in fiber and low in saturated fats, and you'll be well on your way toward reducing your risk of acquiring type 2 diabetes.

Increase Your Longevity and Vitality

Longevity is how long you will live. Vitality is how much energy you have, and how strong and active you are. We all want to live longer and kick butt while doing it. You wouldn't be reading this book if you didn't think so! A CGM is one of your tools to increase your longevity and vitality. If all you ever do after you use a CGM for the next six months or so (I recommend at least six months of use before you'll really understand your glucose responses) is learn to change your diet in a way that reduces your nightly average glucose, while you sleep, and your 24-hour average daily glucose, you'll live longer and have more energy doing it. Just that alone will help prevent cardiovascular disease, stroke, type 2 diabetes, and the healthy diet change that you'll ultimately have to do to lower those numbers will also help prevent cancer. Repeat after me: "Fast food is not healthy!" Cutting the crap foods out of your life, such as junk foods, seed oils, fast food, and foods that "blow up" your blood glucose, are changes that will result in improvements in your metabolism and athletic performance. You'll live even longer—and kick butt doing it! No, a CGM is not the fountain of youth, but it can keep you accountable to your diet and help you to make better choices. Every choice counts. It's you that must make the right choices in your diet, and using a CGM will help you to make those choices and in turn increase your longevity and vitality.

CHAPTER 1

What Is a CGM?

CONTINUOUS GLUCOSE MONITORS (CGMS) are medical devices that measure the continuous interstitial glucose across 24-hour periods.[7] CGM technology enables you to see interstitial glucose responses to dietary intake, carbohydrate ingestion, and physical activity. This sends your glucose data to a compatible smartphone, watch, or bike computer so that you can see it any time you like. Because you sleep with it on as well, it can give you important information about your nighttime glucose levels, which can be impacted by dietary intake. CGMs have been used since 2016 by type 1 and 2 diabetics in the management of diabetes mellitus, providing critical information that allows them to easily respond to glucose fluctuations on an as needed basis.[8]

Currently, and in the past, glucose data has been collected either via self-monitoring with a finger-stick glucometer after a meal or throughout the day, to assess glucose status and administer insulin if needed. Measuring your glucose with a finger stick after your meal makes it challenging to understand exactly your personal response to your meal. Your glucose will be different if you take the measurement 10 minutes after, 12 minutes after, or 20 minutes after, as your body is constantly trying to regulate your glucose after a meal. However, CGMs can report every minute, some every five minutes, while others only report when you scan them with your smartphone. These are accumulated averages over that time period. With the truly *continuous* glucose monitors, you'll learn how your recent food intake and exercise impacted your glucose, giving you an opportunity to adjust insulin dosing (if you are type 1 or 2) and see the impact of your meals or snacks in almost real time. Using a CGM is a truly revolutionary way to measure glucose levels and has been well proven to compare with highly calibrated venous sampling in nondiabetic individuals.[9] Since CGM devices measure interstitial glucose rather than actual blood glucose concentrations, a 5 to 10 minute lag exists between actual blood glucose and reported CGM glucose readings.[10] This is important to remember when you're competing, and we'll talk more about this in later chapters.

HOW TO USE A CGM

CGMs contain a thin sensor that is inserted into the subcutaneous tissue, which could be the back of the upper arm or abdominal wall, or even your upper buttocks. It needs to be in a somewhat "fatty" tissue area, otherwise it will irritate the muscle. This sensor is a glucose-oxidase soaked electrode that measures the glucose level in the interstitial fluid by catalyzing the glucose oxidase reaction, which produces a tiny electrical current that equates to the concentration of glucose in the interstitial fluid. See Figure 1.0. The glucose level is an estimation based upon an algorithm used by the manufacturers of each CGM. Depending on the size of the battery and the type of CGM, they can last from 3 to 14 days (the most common length of time they last) and even up to six months.[11]

Calibration

Many CGMs are calibrated at the factory, but some can be calibrated by using a finger-stick glucometer. Once calibrated, these don't seem to need to be recalibrated, although if you feel like your glucose numbers are too low or too high, I encourage you to recalibrate. Sometimes the CGMs can go "bad," lose connection, fail completely, or begin to read inaccurately. In this case, remove the sensor and apply a new one. For sensors that begin reading low (the most common issue) and are not calibratable, this is a frustrating and deceiving issue. You might think, "Oh, wow, my glucose is really low right now." But, in reality, it's just the sensor itself. A study in 2016 found that calibratable sensors needed to be calibrated between one to four times a day.[12] The calibration is done by the CGM app. In some cases, like with the Abbott's Libre Sense Glucose Sport Biosensor, the sensor can lose the calibration in the Abbott app. However, if you

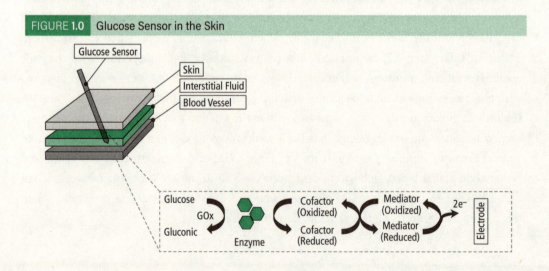

FIGURE 1.0   Glucose Sensor in the Skin

use a third party app, like UltraHuman, then you can calibrate it in their app and prevent wasting a sensor.

Although the technology has come a long way in four years, I have found that you might need to calibrate the sensor an hour or so after insertion, and then one more time the next day. Use your best judgment here, and when in doubt, calibrate it or change out the sensor. Figures 1.1, 1.2, and 1.3 show a comparison between the Abbott's Libre Sense Glucose Sport Biosensor, the Dexcom G7, and a glucometer measurement from a finger stick, all taken simultaneously.

As you can see, they're all different! Reminder: the finger stick is measuring actual blood glucose at your fingertip, whereas the CGM is measuring the glucose in the interstitial fluid, which could lag 5 to 10 minutes behind. If we measured it in your vein directly, we would get yet another different number. The key point here is that they're "consistent" for the non-calibratable CGMs. If it's off by 20 milligrams per deciliter (mg/dL), and as long as it's *always* off

FIGURE 1.1   Finger Stick Accu-Chek—Aviva Glucometer Reading

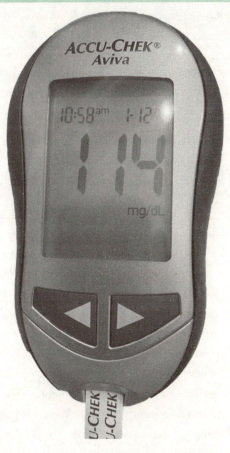

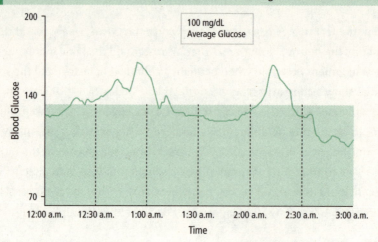

FIGURE 1.2 Abbott's Libre Sense Glucose Sport Biosensor Reading—Not a Calibratable Sensor

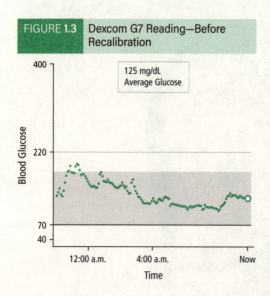

FIGURE 1.3 Dexcom G7 Reading—Before Recalibration

by 20 mg/dL, then that's fine. If it becomes inconsistent and it's off by 5 mg/dL in the morning when your glucose is 75 mg/dL, and then it's off by 30 mg/dL when your blood glucose is 150 mg/dL, that's a problem. So be sure to take a few measurements at different glucose levels to ensure it's consistent.

All CGMs contain a small battery inside them that will only last 3 to 14 days. When they expire a new CGM is required (or you can replace the battery for those that have replaceable batteries). The information is sent to a smartphone via low-energy Bluetooth and can then be sent to smartwatches or bicycle computers. Depending on which CGM you're using, the glucose data can be sent continuously, every one to five minutes, along with synching to your phone automatically, or you might have to do a "manual swipe" using the back of your phone to swipe over the sensor, sending the data to your CGM app. A manual swipe is less useful to be certain, especially if you're in a competition. If you do lose connection with your phone, or let's say you leave your phone in another room, then the CGM will store average readings every five minutes for up to eight hours. The next time you reconnect your smartphone, the information will download from the CGM. You'll notice right away that the glucose line is smoother and less jagged than normal. This is because of the lower frequency of measurements being saved vs. being sent continuously. This also means that you could lose a lot of important data in that smoothed line. The smartphone CGM app is truly where the CGM goes from being a "tech gadget" to a useful tool. All the manufacturers of CGMs produce their own smartphone apps, and there are many third-party apps that allow a deeper dive into your glucose levels over time. You can view this data in real time and retrospectively to help you better understand trends, patterns, and how your glucose levels change quickly or more slowly. I encourage you to also record your meals if your app has that capability. For instance, the Levels app has the ability for you to use voice-to-text and allows you to speak "natural language" so it can analyze what you're saying and then categorize it as separate foods. This is very, very handy! Most companies also have a web application, which allows you to further analyze your data.

CGMS AND APPS

There are many CGMs on the market and most of them require a prescription from a doctor. Abbott Labs, Dexcom, Eversense, Medtronic, GlucoMen in Europe, and other companies all make CGMs for use by type 1 and 2 diabetics. In 2024, the US Food and Drug Administration (FDA) approved multiple sensors for use by consumers without a doctor's prescription. These are the sensors from Dexcom Stelo, Abbott Labs Lingo, and Libre Rio. This list will continue to grow and it's likely that more have been approved since the writing and publication of this book. The sensors continue to evolve, by improving in accuracy, battery level, and simplicity of application.

CGMs have their own proprietary apps to view and use the information they gather. These all work on your smartphone and are relatively simple and easy to use. As with any software, there are pluses and minuses to each app, for example relating to the number of features and how useful the metrics are. These companies make their apps relatively simple for the common denominator end-user and don't care much about improving them beyond the basic features. These apps are also very diabetic-centric and less about improving overall health—and certainly not about athletic performance. This has created an opportunity for other software companies to come in, create their own apps that work with the CGM sensor directly (via Bluetooth signal) or piggyback off a manufacturer's app, essentially hijacking the information. Most of these third-party apps are also more focused on health than athletic performance, therefore, providing a much richer feature set, including some incredibly innovative metrics, food logging, trend analysis, and even predictive glucose values based on their dataset. There are a couple of apps that are integrating AI capabilities to leverage their entire user database of foods and glucose responses to help you make better decisions. This area is incredibly exciting, and we'll only continue to see improvements over time. Unfortunately, in mid-2024, the main company focused on athletic performance, Supersapiens, went out of business, largely due to the FDA dragging its heels in approving the Abbott's Libre Sense Glucose Sport Biosensor. Supersapiens—founded by Phil Southerland, former pro cyclist (also a type 1 diabetic) and founder of the Team Type 1 cycling team—and its app really created some outstanding features for athletes. It's a real shame they could no longer continue, and my hope is that they'll return with renewed vigor. That being said, other companies are producing apps that will be highly useful for athletes, and I expect we'll continue to see this area grow very quickly in the coming years. The main third-party apps available in the market, at the time of publishing are:

- www.levelshealth.com
- www.ultrahuman.com
- www.veri.co
- www.nutrisense.io

These all have features that are incredibly useful for the athlete, with UltraHuman and Levels leading the charge.

WHAT IS BLOOD GLUCOSE?

Blood glucose, or blood sugar, is a critical component of human physiology. It serves as a primary source of energy, especially for the brain and muscles, and plays an integral role in maintaining overall health. Blood glucose is the concentration of glucose (a simple sugar) present in the bloodstream. When we ingest carbohydrates, we convert those carbohydrates into glucose molecules. These molecules can be used immediately and are stored in the liver and/or muscles as glycogen. They can also be stored as fat if we eat too many calories and have an excess of glucose.

It's important to know a few key terms related to blood glucose as you read the rest of this book.

Hypoglycemia

Hypoglycemia occurs when blood glucose levels fall below normal and is usually considered below 70 mg/dL. It is often referred to as "low blood sugar," and can result from prolonged fasting, intense exercise, or certain medical conditions. Symptoms of hypoglycemia can include shakiness, sweating, rapid heartbeat, and, in severe cases, confusion, seizures, or coma. As an athlete, a sudden drop in blood glucose during prolonged exercise is known as "bonking" or "hitting the wall," which severely impairs performance. So read that sentence again. *A sudden drop* is the key descriptor. Dr. Stephen McGregor, professor of exercise physiology at Eastern Michigan University said, "You don't have a bonk just because you drop below 70 mg/dL. You can bonk if you're used to a high level of blood glucose and then that drops a certain amount. You could be competing with a glucose from 140 to 180 mg/dL for hours and hours, and then you drop to 120 mg/dL. You could experience all the symptoms of hypoglycemia, and your performance will be severely impacted. A big part of your performance is your body's perception and the level of glucose you are accustomed to. When you're accustomed to being hyperglycemic, then when that level drops dramatically, you experience the bonk."[13]

Hyperglycemia

Hyperglycemia, the opposite of hypoglycemia (low blood glucose), refers to having elevated blood glucose levels. This is generally thought to be over 126 mg/dL during fasting and over 180 mg/dL two hours after your meal. The glucose level for hyperglycemia hasn't been determined yet for nondiabetic athletes during exercise, as using CGMs for non-diabetics is so new. I have found in over two years of researching across 12 different sports that athletes can compete at a high level with their glucose at 200 mg/dL or greater. So in non-diabetics, during exercise, hyperglycemia might be considered over 200 mg/dL, but this is only an observation at this point. More research is needed.

Hyperglycemia can be caused by factors such as excessive carbohydrate intake, insulin resistance, or insufficient insulin production. From a health perspective, chronic hyperglycemia is a sign of diabetes and can lead to long-term complications such as cardiovascular disease, kidney damage, blindness, stroke, neuropathy, and ultimately death. As an athlete, it's fine to have a high glucose level during exercise, but you want to have a lower, more "normal," level during the rest of your life.

Glycogen

Glycogen is the stored form of glucose, primarily found in the liver and muscles. It serves as a readily available energy reserve that can be quickly mobilized when blood glucose levels drop or during periods of increased energy demand, such as training and/or competition. The main difference between glycogen and glucose is that glycogen is a polysaccharide, meaning it consists of multiple glucose molecules linked together, whereas glucose is a monosaccharide, a single sugar molecule. Glycogen levels are very important to you as an athlete, and they have a significant impact on athletic performance. Through training and "carbo-loading," you can increase your muscle's ability to store more glycogen. And with high glycogen stores, you can sustain longer periods of intense exercise before fatiguing. Conversely, low glycogen levels can lead to early fatigue and decreased performance.

Trained athletes have roughly a total of two and a half hours of stored glycogen in their muscles and liver. In the muscles, there can be as much as two hours of stored glycogen (300 g) in highly trained athletes and 30 minutes of stored glycogen (100 g) in the liver, so elite athletes could have up to around two and a half hours of stored glycogen. For recreational athletes, this could be only one and a half hours of stored glycogen, so there could be a vast difference between recreational and elite professionals.[14]

Glycogenesis

Glycogenesis is the process by which glucose is converted into glycogen for storage in the liver and muscles. This process happens when there is an excess of glucose in the bloodstream, such as after a meal. What this means is that this process is taking the glucose out of the bloodstream and reducing your glucose number on your CGM. Glycogenesis is also crucial for maintaining blood glucose levels within a normal range and for ensuring that the body has sufficient energy reserves for future use.

Glycolysis

Glycolysis is a fundamental energy-producing process in cells, converting glucose into pyruvate while generating adenosine triphosphate (ATP). This is the first step in cellular respiration and occurs in the cytoplasm of cells. In other words, this is the "burning of glucose" to help create energy in your body. Glycolysis is particularly important during high-intensity anaerobic exercise when the demand for energy exceeds the supply of oxygen, as it can produce ATP quickly without the need for oxygen. This means that if you're doing very intense but short exercise, like a sprint on the track, a lift on the bench press, or anything maximal effort that is less than 60 seconds, you're calling on the glycolysis process for energy.

Glycogenolysis

Glycogenolysis is the process of breaking down glycogen into glucose, which can then be released into the bloodstream or used by muscles for energy. All that stored glycogen must be broken back down into glucose for use. This process happens during periods of fasting, stress, or intense exercise when blood glucose levels begin to drop. According to Dr. Andrew R. Coggan, the author of several papers on the subject, "At the onset of exercise, the rate of glycogenolysis accelerates to match hepatic (liver) glucose output to increased peripheral (mostly muscle) glucose uptake, so it will dominate initially. As time (minutes to hours, not seconds to minutes) goes by, hepatic (liver) glycogenolysis gradually decreases (as glycogen stores become depleted), with gluconeogenesis having to increase to take up the slack."[15] Glycogenolysis ensures that the body has a continuous steady supply of glucose, even when dietary intake is insufficient.

Gluconeogenesis

What happens when you deplete all your glycogen stores, and you don't ingest more glucose? That's when your body's back-up system kicks in. This is called gluconeogenesis and is the process of producing glucose from non-carbohydrate sources, such as proteins (amino acids), lactate, and fats (glycerol). This process primarily occurs in the liver and is essential during prolonged fasting, starvation, or intense exercise when glycogen stores are depleted. Gluconeogenesis helps maintain blood glucose levels and provides energy to organs that rely heavily on glucose, such as the brain. Your body will protect your brain at all costs from starving from lack of glucose. It goes so far as to shut down the rest of your body to preserve your brain. You won't be able to walk and will collapse from fatigue, a direct result of your body protecting your brain and ensuring it has glucose to survive.

POWERING THE BODY

Glucose itself is not the direct fuel that powers the body. Instead, glucose is used to make ATP, the true energy source for all the body's cells. Here's how it works in the simplest of explanations.

It begins with ingestion and digestion. You eat foods that contain carbohydrates, which are then broken down into simpler sugars, primarily glucose, in the digestive system. Next comes absorption and transportation of that glucose. This is what we are measuring with a CGM: the actual transportation of the glucose to the interstitial fluid (fatty layer part of your skin). The glucose is then absorbed into the bloodstream and moved to cells throughout the body. Here's where insulin comes in. When you eat food and that food is broken down into glucose and then enters the bloodstream, this will send a specific signal to the pancreas to release insulin. Insulin "opens the door" for the uptake of glucose into cells, particularly muscle and liver cells.

Once inside the cells, this is where ATP is produced. Glucose goes through multiple processes, which you might remember from high school biology class. Some light biochemistry here!

1. **Glycolysis**: Glucose is broken down into pyruvate, producing a small amount of ATP (two molecules) and nicotinamide adenine dinucleotide (NADH) (another energy-carrying molecule).

2. **Krebs Cycle**: Pyruvate enters the mitochondria (the engine of the cell) and is further processed, generating more NADH and flavin adenine dinucleotide (FADH2) (another energy carrier).

3. **Oxidative Phosphorylation (Electron Transport Chain)**: NADH and FADH2 are used to generate a large amount of ATP (28 molecules) through a process that involves the transfer of electrons and the creation of a proton gradient.

After all that happens, those precious energy molecules of ATP are used to power many of your cells' activities, and as an athlete, that ATP is critical for muscle contraction, transmission of nerve signals and other biochemical reactions that will help you to perform at your best. So, while glucose is essential because it's the primary source of fuel for ATP production, it's ATP that fuels the body's activities.

And here's the information you've been waiting for, and why this all matters: without sufficient glucose, cells wouldn't be able to produce the necessary ATP to function effectively, leading to a decline in overall athletic performance. Our muscles, brain, and liver are particularly dependent on blood glucose.

How does this impact more specifically the muscles, brain, and liver? When we exercise, train and/or compete, our muscles require a tremendous amount of energy. Most of the energy used by the muscles is in the form of stored glycogen, but those stores must be in the muscles to be used. However, if needed, glucose can be rapidly taken up by muscle cells and converted into ATP through glycolysis. This process provides the immediate energy needed for muscle contraction.

The brain is the most glucose-dependent organ in the body. Unlike muscles, which can also use fat for energy, the brain relies almost exclusively on glucose (it can also use ketones, supplied or made by the body). A constant supply of glucose is necessary to maintain cognitive functions, such as thinking, memory, and learning. One of the first signs of low blood glucose is the lack of ability to think clearly.

Finally, the liver acts as a glucose storage unit, or gas tank so to speak, storing glucose in the form of glycogen. When blood glucose levels drop, the liver releases glucose back into the bloodstream through a process called glycogenolysis. The liver also plays a role in gluconeogenesis, which is the production of glucose from non-carbohydrate sources (proteins and fats), which ensures a steady supply of glucose during fasting or prolonged exercise. So yes, you can exercise just on proteins and fats, but this must be at a low level of intensity. In the book *Sport Nutrition*, Dr. Asker Jeukendrup and Dr. Michael Gleeson wrote, "The main problem with the use of fat as a fuel for exercise is the rate at which it can be taken up by muscle and oxidized to provide energy. Fat oxidation can only supply ATP at a rate sufficient to maintain exercise at an intensity of about 60% of V̇O2max."[16]

INSULIN

Now that you understand the glucose side of the equation, you also need to know a few things about insulin.

Insulin is a peptide hormone which is produced by the beta cells in the pancreas. This happens as a response to increased glucose levels, typically after eating.[17] It is essential for controlling blood glucose levels and ensuring that cells receive the energy they need to function. Insulin can be thought of as the "key to unlocking the door" to the cells, which allows glucose, proteins, and nutrients to enter the cells. And when the glucose enters the cells, it leaves the bloodstream, thereby lowering your blood glucose.

As soon as you put some glucose in your mouth, insulin begins secreting and stops the fat burning process (lipolysis). Once glucose enters the bloodstream from the digestive system, insulin acts like a key, unlocking cells so they can absorb glucose. And if you just read about the process of the Krebs cycle in the Powering the Body section above, you'll know that the glucose can then be converted into ATP or stored as glycogen for later use, particularly in the liver and muscles. It's also very important to understand that your body also secretes insulin when you eat proteins and fats. This is important to understand the implications regarding a high protein/high fat diet as many believe that by reducing the glucose spikes by abstaining from carbs, they're avoiding any future issues with regards to type 2 diabetes. This is flawed thinking and will be detailed in Chapter 7.

If you eat too much food, or more than you expend, insulin also promotes the storage of excess glucose as fat in adipose tissue (fat). It's worth repeating that insulin inhibits the breakdown of fat and glycogen, helping to maintain energy balance in the body. What does this mean to you as an athlete? If you're trying to reduce your fat percentage by cutting out calories and fasting, then keep in mind that as soon as you put carbs in your mouth, that fat burning process is stopped. If you don't produce insulin like a type 1 diabetic (who has to inject insulin), glucose would remain in the bloodstream, causing hyperglycemia (high blood glucose), which has been proven to cause a range of health issues, including damage to blood vessels, nerves, and organs. That damage then leads to cardiovascular damage, a possible heart attack, and even death. So, insulin is very important, along with a well-functioning pancreas!

Without insulin, the body's ability to regulate blood glucose levels is severely compromised, leading to hyperglycemia. If left untreated, this condition can result in serious health complications, including diabetic ketoacidosis (DKA), a life-threatening condition where the body begins to break down fat for energy, producing high levels of ketones and leading to acidic blood. People with type 1 diabetes, a condition where the pancreas produces little to no insulin, require external insulin administration to manage their blood glucose levels. Without insulin treatment, individuals with type 1 diabetes would not survive. Even in type 2 diabetes, where the body becomes resistant to insulin, the importance of insulin remains, as the condition can lead to similar complications if not properly managed.

Unfortunately, there is no continuous insulin monitor as this would be just as interesting as a CGM and very possibly even more helpful to the athlete. Insulin is the opposite side of the "same coin" and we have to infer what is happening with insulin through the monitoring of glucose. We can come close to understanding this but, still, it's an imprecise estimate.

Besides the immediate risks of hyperglycemia, a lack of insulin would also mean that cells could not efficiently absorb glucose, leading to severe energy deficits. The brain, which relies almost exclusively on glucose for energy, would be particularly affected, resulting in cognitive impairment, confusion, and, in extreme cases, coma. This is what happens when someone enters a diabetic coma. Without insulin, the body's ability to store energy in the form of glycogen and fat would be severely impaired, leading to rapid weight loss, muscle wasting, and malnutrition. In the long term, chronic hyperglycemia without insulin management can cause irreversible damage to various organs, leading to complications such as blindness, kidney failure, and cardiovascular disease.

Insulin Sensitivity vs. Insulin Resistance

Insulin sensitivity is what you want as an athlete and in life. Insulin sensitivity is how responsive the body's cells are to insulin. High insulin sensitivity means cells readily respond to insulin's signal to absorb glucose from the bloodstream. This is a good thing! You want that glucose level to come down quickly. Individuals with high insulin sensitivity require less insulin to manage blood glucose levels, which is generally a sign of good metabolic health. The great news is that through exercising; eating a healthy diet full of fruit and vegetables and fiber, and low in saturated fat; and maintaining a healthy weight, you can improve your insulin sensitivity.

Insulin resistance occurs when the body's cells become less responsive to insulin, meaning more and more insulin is required to achieve the same effect. As a result, the pancreas compensates by producing more insulin, leading to elevated insulin levels (hyperinsulinemia). Over time, this can exhaust the pancreas and lead to conditions such as type 2 diabetes. Insulin resistance is what you're trying to prevent in athletic events and in your everyday life. Reducing high sugar intake, ultra-processed foods, saturated fats, sedentary periods, and keeping your weight down, will help reduce insulin resistance.

What about the role exercise plays here? Before exercise, insulin helps ensure that muscles have sufficient glycogen stores by promoting glucose uptake and glycogenesis (the conversion of glucose to glycogen). This glycogen serves as a readily available energy source during exercise. During exercise, insulin levels naturally decrease to allow for the mobilization of glucose and fatty acids from storage sites. This process is essential for maintaining blood glucose levels and providing a steady energy supply to working muscles. After exercise, insulin sensitivity temporarily increases, meaning cells are highly responsive to insulin's effects. This heightened sensitivity allows for post-workout shakes and meals to be quickly metabolized and the glucose to be taken up in the muscles and liver quicker, enhancing your post-workout recovery. Therefore, you *want* a glucose spike after your workout. That recovery shake, containing carbs and some protein, that you ingested is important because it causes as much insulin to release as possible, so you can optimize this recovery process aiding in muscle repair and growth.[18]

THE THREE MAIN FACTORS THAT INFLUENCE BLOOD GLUCOSE READINGS IN CGMS

Movement

Exercise is your biggest tool to reduce your circulating blood glucose. When your glucose is high, go for a brisk walk, ride your bike, do some work in the gym, play racquetball, or anything else to get you moving. The carbohydrates you ingest will be turned into glucose and start circulating in the bloodstream. Your body prioritizes using those carbohydrates as fuel first before requiring the breakdown of glycogen from the liver into glucose (glycogenolysis). This is great for endurance athletes, as it helps to preserve your liver and muscle glycogen during the first two-thirds of a competition and saves those precious glycogen stores for the last third of competitions. If you don't use this circulating glucose, then you'll either store it in the liver or muscles as glycogen (glycogenesis) or store it as fat to be used during very low-intensity workouts—or during famine or the apocalypse.

For your purposes, you need to always remember that if you start exercising, your glucose level will most likely drop, especially if it's just an easy- to moderate-intensity workout. If it's a low-intensity workout, you'll burn mostly fat. However, a very low-intensity workout, like a walk after dinner, will cause your glucose to drop since your body will prioritize this readily available source of energy. This drop in glucose is normal, so don't be surprised when you see it occur. In most cases, your glucose will drop but then come back up to normal level as your body finds an equilibrium between the supply of blood glucose and the demand from the muscles. If your glucose value is already on the low side of your normal level, then exercise will drop it even more and your liver will begin releasing glycogen into the bloodstream to take up the slack. If your glucose level is on the high side after a heavy carbohydrate meal, then exercising will reduce the level of glucose in your bloodstream, which is a good thing. In Figure 1.4, an athlete does just that. A heavy-carb meal, with a big increase in glucose, followed by a 30-minute brisk walk brings the glucose level right back down.

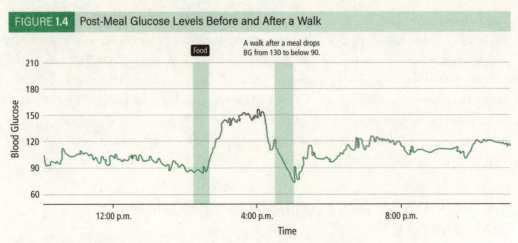

After eating a carb-heavy meal, going for a walk can bring down glucose levels.

Nutrition

This one should be obvious. What you eat has a massive influence on your glucose levels. If you eat only protein, then your glucose level will barely budge. If you eat only fats, your glucose levels will barely budge. You need glucose in your system to be able to measure it. When you ingest sugars, whether a simple sugar like fructose or a complex sugar like starch, they're going to raise your glucose. How much you ingest of each type will determine the height of the peak of your glucose, and your metabolic efficiency will determine how quickly it drops or stays up. It's not always that cut and dried though, as the height and length of the peak is also determined by the fiber content, protein amount, and fat amount in your food. This combines to determine your glucose level. To make it even more complicated, what you had in your previous meal and your current training status can also impact your glucose response. Overall, though, what you put in your mouth has a large influence on your glucose levels. As we saw in Figure 1.4, a high-carbohydrate meal can send your blood glucose through the roof. In Figure 1.5, we have an athlete that has a normal glucose level while sleeping, down around 90 mg/dL. He then gets up and has a high-carbohydrate breakfast, which spikes his glucose to nearly 180 mg/dL, before it begins to dissipate. At lunch time, he goes out for a meal at a Mexican restaurant. He indulges in some chips; a large burrito filled with beans, rice, and veggies; and finishes it off with four small chocolates back at the office. This sends his glucose value to 200 mg/dL, possibly higher, and keeps it there for over four hours! Clearly, this athlete didn't need this much fuel on board.

Mood

Excitement, nervousness, anticipation, anxiousness, stress, and fear are moods/feelings that can raise your blood glucose. These feelings (and others) can release adrenalin (epinephrine),

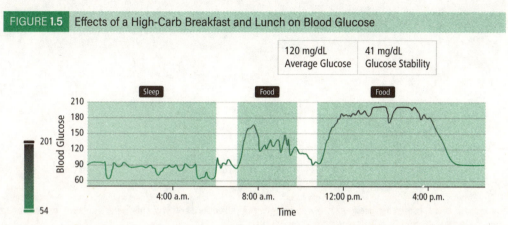

Eating an excessive amount of calories when not needed can cause your glucose to rise and stay elevated.

which causes the stimulation of glycogen breakdown in the liver and fat burning in the fatty (adipose) tissue (lipolysis). Anytime you trigger the sense of "fight or flight," adrenalin is released, and glucose is released into the bloodstream to deal with the threat. Your body doesn't know if it's about to be chased by a bear or if you're just getting ready for a big presentation at work! Technically, this is a reaction in the sympathetic nervous system, which prepares the body for this fight or flight, whereas the parasympathetic nervous system restores the body to a calm and relaxed state. So yes, if your glucose shoots up right before a big presentation at work, it's not an error. It's a real release of glucose so that you have the energy you need to "wow" the boss. That also can happen in a heated argument, when you're excited for an upcoming event, are nervous before a big competition, or feel stressed by a tough situation. Your mood absolutely influences your glucose levels. So, if you're watching your numbers and you see them go up and wonder why, think back to your mood and see if that was the cause.

In Figure 1.6, we see an athlete that has a big presentation at work causing a significant increase in glucose. The sympathetic system kicks in and signals to the liver to begin releasing glycogen and turning that into glucose for energy.

WHAT DOES THIS ALL MEAN TO YOU?

This is complicated stuff. Just like how I don't know how my cell phone works—what all the transistors, chips, signals, etc. are—I know when I pick up the phone, I can call someone around the world instantly. You don't need to know every single detail about the biochemistry behind your glucose value being measured on your CGM. What's important to know while reading this book and observing your glucose levels on your CGM, is that *your* glucose response is based on many factors. There is no absolute, where Y always equals mx+b, in glucose monitoring.

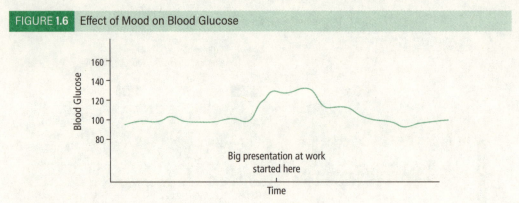

FIGURE 1.6 Effect of Mood on Blood Glucose

Your mood can cause your glucose to rise. Adrenalin can be released when you are excited, stressed, or threatened, which results in glucose being released into the bloodstream.

Mood, movement, and nutrition are the big factors. Within nutrition, there is timing, type of food, state of fasting, fat-burning state, and more. If you've just eaten a large meal that was 60% carbs, 30% protein, and 10% fat, followed by a brisk hour-long walk, you might see a drop in your glucose because you were using all those circulating sugars you ingested at dinner. How about being in a 16-hour fasted state and then eating three donuts for breakfast? You might get a spike in glucose that goes over 200 mg/dL vs. if you eat those same three donuts at the end of a normal day where you're eating every three hours or so.

There's mood to consider as well. If you're preparing for a big presentation at work, but haven't eaten since breakfast, just the excitement of the presentation can cause your liver to release glucose into your bloodstream and raise your glucose, despite not having any food for over four hours. What happens to your mood when your glucose level is dropping? Maybe you notice you're not in a very good mood for some reason or the other and then realize that your glucose level has been dropping slowly over four hours and is now at 65 mg/dL.

Movement impacts your glucose levels dramatically, whether you're going for an easy walk after dinner or doing VO2 max hill repeats on the local trail. The spike that comes from intense exercise can turn into a slow downward drop as you use your glycogen stores and circulating glucose, which makes it so important to understand when you need to ingest more food to stay ahead of the drop. An easy walk after your dinner is something that I highly encourage, as very low-intensity exercise helps to reduce the circulating glucose that you just ingested from dinner and helps to keep your nightly average glucose lower.

In the coming chapters, you'll continue to learn more about what the graphs and charts from CGM data mean, how you can apply this data in your own training and competition, and how your body responds.

| | CHAPTER 2 |

How Foods Impact Your Glucose and Performance

IT'S DIFFICULT TO BE CERTAIN ABOUT the impact of different foods on your performance. The responses to foods can be wildly different from one person to another. One person might have oatmeal with strawberries, flax, a tablespoon of almond butter, and almond milk for their breakfast and barely get glucose rising from 80 milligrams per deciliter (mg/dL) to 90 mg/dL, and they might not be able to get a spike throughout the whole day. Another person might have the same small meal and get a fast spike that sends them from 80 mg/dL to 150 mg/dL. The same meal and proportions but vastly different responses. The cause of this is multifactorial and hard to blame on any one component. It could be related to your meal the night before, the intensity of your training the day before, how depleted (or not) your glycogen stores are, the quality of your sleep, individual physiological factors, the level of stress you're exposed to, and even your age. It could also be related to the drugs you're taking. Keep in mind that other chronic medical conditions and/or the therapy you're taking might interfere with your glucose levels/trends.

What's important to understand for you, are the responses that you receive on average or as a trend. As you read this chapter, you'll see examples and case studies of different athletes and their glucose responses. This will help to give you a clearer understanding of how your daily foods, training and post-workout nutrition, and recovery strategies, all play a role in improving your performance in the pool, the gym, the bike, or whatever sport you engage in. Make sure to keep an open mind as you read this chapter, and also remind yourself that these examples are of one person on one day. It may or may not apply to you, but I hope that I've included enough different examples that you'll be able to make better decisions in your food choices, not only for performance reasons but also for your long-term health and longevity.

SIMPLE AND COMPLEX CARBOHYDRATES

Simple carbohydrates (or simple sugars) consist of basic sugar molecules (short chain). They're quickly digested and absorbed by the body. When you think of simple carbs, think quick energy and rapid increases in blood glucose. Some examples of these are fruits (fructose) and dairy products (lactose). Simple carbs are also commonly added to foods, such as table sugar, corn syrup, and high-fructose corn syrup. What are common foods that have simple carbs? Soda, baked treats like cookies and pies, packaged cookies, fruit juice concentrate like orange juice, and breakfast cereals. Simple carbs are hidden in many foods as well, including salad dressings, sandwich bread, and yogurt.

Complex carbohydrates or complex sugars have longer chains of sugar molecules. They take longer to digest and provide more stable energy. When you think of complex carbohydrates, think of more sustained blood glucose levels, still giving you a rise in blood glucose but not such a tall spike, yet the rise might last longer. Hence the overall glucose response might seem more stable. Some common examples of complex carbs include: whole grains (e.g., brown rice, quinoa, and oats); legumes (e.g., beans and lentils); vegetables; fruits (with fiber); and some starchy foods (e.g., potatoes and whole-grain bread). Notice anything different about this list than the simple carb list? Yes, complex carbs are more whole plant-based foods that contain fiber, not processed foods that have been stripped of their fiber. Fiber helps to slow the digestion of the sugars in the plants and, therefore, mute the spike in glucose levels. Moreover, "epidemiological and clinical studies demonstrate that intake of dietary fiber and whole grain is inversely related to obesity, type two diabetes, cancer and cardiovascular disease (CVD)."[19]

What about high-glycemic and low-glycemic foods? When we talk about simple and complex carbs, it's also important to clearly understand the Glycemic Index (GI) and how that relates to your blood glucose. Are all simple carbs high glycemic? Are all complex carbs low glycemic? The GI is a metric that ranks your carbohydrate intake based on post-meal glucose responses in comparison to the "gold" standard of pure glucose, which scores 100 on the GI. Foods that are higher on the index contain more sugars and, therefore, produce a higher blood glucose level. Foods that are lower on the GI have less sugars and consequently cause a lower glucose level or possibly no rise at all.[20] Therefore, the GI is a way to rank foods containing carbs on a scale from 1 to 100 based on how much they affect your blood sugar levels. Two foods with the same amount of carbohydrates can have different GI numbers, so just because you eat a gel with 100 kilocalories (k/cals), doesn't mean it will give you the same glucose response as eating a sports bar with 100 k/cals.

Foods are grouped into three categories based on their GI: low, medium, and high. A score of 100 means that a food has a big effect on your glucose levels (and insulin), while a score of

CHAPTER 2: How Foods Impact Your Glucose and Performance   19

one indicates little effect. GI can help you make better sports-nutrition choices based on what you need at the time. Maybe you're about to start a bike race and you want to "prime" your body for the start, so you want to eat something that'll give you a quick spike just 10 minutes before you begin. In this case, you would choose a high-glycemic food, which usually means more processed, simple carbs and less or no fiber. On the other hand, you could be at hour five of a full-distance triathlon and know that you've five more hours to go, so a lower-glycemic food would be more appropriate to give you a slower release for longer-term energy. Here's the GI ranking:[21]

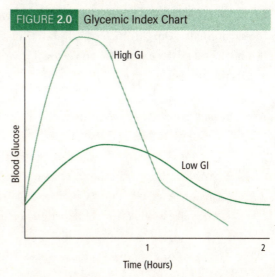

High-glycemic foods result in a quick spike in insulin and blood sugar (also known as blood glucose). Low-glycemic foods have a slower, smaller effect.

1–55 = Low
56–69 = Medium

The reason some foods make glucose shoot up fast, is that simple carbohydrates in them, such as refined sugars and white flour, are easier for your body to change into glucose (the sugar your body uses for energy) as these are short-chain sugars and quickly broken down. In contrast, carbs such as those in vegetables and whole grains are digested more slowly, as mentioned earlier, as complex carbs with fiber and more long-chain molecules take longer for the body to break down. If you eat lower-glycemic foods, it will be easier to regulate your blood glucose and keep your energy levels more stable for a longer period. If you eat a lot of high-GI carbs, you may have a harder time controlling your blood sugar and could quickly put yourself on a "roller coaster" glucose response, which we'll talk about in later chapters.

You need glucose, and in the right amount, to enhance your athletic performance, whether that's during training or a competition. Making sure that you take in just the right type of carbs at the right time will make the difference between feeling energized and ready to go at the start, or lethargic and ready for a nap. Your body makes hormones to control glucose levels. These hormones include insulin and glucagon. "Insulin potentially coordinates with glucagon to modulate blood glucose levels; insulin acts via an anabolic pathway, while glucagon performs catabolic functions."[22] Insulin moves glucose from your blood into your other organs.

Glucagon releases glucose stored in your liver when you need more blood sugar. Your body should normally keep glucose levels at a healthy level. I'll elaborate more on insulin throughout this book and by the end of the book, you'll have a clear understanding of how insulin works and its role in performance.

Examples of low-GI foods include:
- Green vegetables and raw carrots.
- Legumes like lentils, black beans, kidney beans, soybeans, pinto beans, etc.
- Nuts like almonds, walnuts, cashews, peanuts, etc.
- Unsweetened plant milks, non-fat unsweetened yogurt, and milk.
- Fruits like blackberries, blueberries, grapes, oranges, apples, pears, etc.

Examples of medium-GI foods include:
- Vegetables like corn and beets.
- Fruits like figs, bananas, pineapple, and cherries.
- Most dried fruits like raisins, apples, figs, and cranberries.
- Unsweetened whole cereals and most cereals containing whole oats.
- Long grain rice, brown rice, pasta, barley, rice noodles, and couscous.
- Honey and real maple syrup.
- Many breads containing multigrain and nuts, whole-grain wheat, and rye, as well as some sourdough breads.

Examples of high-GI foods include:
- Pure table sugar.
- Risotto, white rice, sticky rice and rice cakes.
- Bagels, white bread and most crackers.
- Cooked carrots and baked or boiled potatoes.
- Doughnuts, candies and chocolates.
- Fruits like watermelon, and all fruits in canned syrup.
- Sweetened cereals.

What about foods that have different versions of themselves? Potatoes for example. Are they all high glycemic? Well, most are, but some are medium, and you might even eat a low-glycemic one. Which one you choose will most definitely have an impact on your blood glucose. See Figure 2.1.

Can You Change the Glycemic Index of Foods?

The GI is just a measure of the single piece of food in either a raw or cooked state. You can change the GI of many foods based on how you cook the food, store the food, and how you combine it with the other foods on your plate. It can also depend on how ripe that food is. For example, a green banana has a GI of around 30, and a "just beyond" ripe banana has a GI of around 60. The green banana contains more resistant starch and less sugar.

FIGURE **2.1** Glycemic Index of Different Potatoes

Potato Types	Glycemic Index (GI)
Baked russet potato	111
Instant mashed potato	87
Boiled white potato	82
Mashed potato	78
Tater tots	75
Purple potatoes	77
Sweet potato	70
French fries	63
Small baked white potato with skin	50
Yam	54

Cooking and food prep. If you add in fat, other fibers, proteins, and acid (such as lemon juice or vinegar), then you'll lower the GI. By combining a high-glycemic food with other low-glycemic foods, you can easily reduce the glucose spike and peak. For example, eating a salad with vegetables and a simple olive oil and vinegar dressing first, followed by white rice with tofu will help to significantly reduce the blood glucose spike and peak, versus eating the white rice all by itself. Cooking time also impacts the GI and if you cook a lower-glycemic food, like yams, so long that it breaks down the fiber, it will no longer be a lower-glycemic carb. Even pasta, a meal that almost every athlete loves, is susceptible to this. The longer you cook starches, such as pasta, the higher their glycemic index will be. Make sure your pasta is al dente.

Storing your food. Surprising, but true: if you put starchy foods with a higher GI in the refrigerator overnight, straight after cooking them, they'll undergo a chemical reaction causing the starch to become more "resistant." When you eat foods with resistant starch, you can't digest them as easily, which lowers the GI and, in turn, reduces your glucose spike. Resistant starches are one of the latest ways that many bread companies are reducing the number of simple, high-glycemic carbs in their products and producing low-carb breads.

Ripe fruits and veggies. The GI of many fruits, such as figs, pears, raspberries, and blackberries, goes up as they ripen. Unripe fruit or vegetables take longer for your body to digest because they contain more fiber and fewer naturally developed sugars. A ripened fruit or vegetable has had more time to create sugars, by turning fiber into sugar, so it digests more quickly and your glucose will increase faster and peak higher.

With this all in mind, what about fats and proteins? These have a GI of 0, as they contain no carbohydrates, so they don't affect blood glucose levels. It's important to understand that this doesn't mean you should add in tons of fats and proteins to better reduce your blood glucose spikes, because not having a spike is not always the answer. You want the appropriate change in blood glucose for the appropriate training or competition. Repeat after me: "The keto diet is *not* the answer. The keto diet is *not* the answer. The keto diet is *not* the answer." As mentioned in the previous chapter, when you first start using a continuous glucose monitor (CGM), you'll immediately see what foods begin impacting your blood glucose and many of you will freak out and think that you need to stop eating all carbs. This is *not* the answer if you want to improve your athletic performance. You'll learn more about this in specific examples later in this chapter.

Now that you know a little more about simple and complex carbs, and high- and low-glycemic foods, let's go into more depth about the timing of food intake and how this influences your blood glucose.

OPTIMAL TIMING OF FOOD INTAKE

When you eat carbs, proteins, and fats (along with how you eat them and the order in which you eat them) this has an incredible impact on your blood glucose levels and correspondingly your performance. Let's start with the easiest examples and work toward the most complicated. Our first example is that of a bodybuilder that has a high-carbohydrate, medium-glycemic meal about 30 to 40 minutes before an intense session in the weight room. There is very little protein and fat in his meal (less than 15%). It's a truly high-carb meal of day-old pasta with a touch of olive oil, 12 celery sticks dipped in hummus, two slices of Ezekiel bread with almond butter, and a raw apple. In Figure 2.2, notice how his blood glucose rises within 15 minutes of his meal and peaks about 30 minutes after his meal, at about the same time he started his gym session.

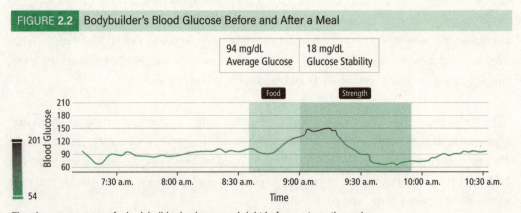

FIGURE 2.2 Bodybuilder's Blood Glucose Before and After a Meal

The glucose response of a bodybuilder having a meal right before a strength session.

(Reminder: the time-to-response is individual and with this kind of meal it will be around 30 minutes to max spike, but it may still vary from athlete to athlete.) Starting from a 90 mg/dL start point and peaking at 140–150 mg/dL at the start of the session, will allow him to start the weight workout with more energy and hopefully accomplish his goals for that session. This is an example of what you want to do before your workout; you want to raise the glucose levels. As you can see in Figure 2.2, as he continues with his workout, his glucose levels lower throughout. This is normal and desired. However, his glucose levels did drop a little lower than I would have preferred at the end of his workout. For the next workout, using a sports drink or having a snack about 45 minutes into the workout would have kept his glucose more stable at the end.

The next example shows how a reactive hypoglycemic crash before a workout can negatively affect the workout. A reactive hypoglycemic crash happens after you ingest carbs—generally simple but can be complex—that cause insulin secretion to rise. If this happens too far in advance of the workout, your body sugar will have already dropped down when your workout starts. Once the workout starts, you'll reduce the glucose levels even more. This combined effect of a higher insulin release with exercise causes the reactive hypoglycemic crash. We'll talk more about reactive hypoglycemic crashes in Chapter 6, including how to prevent them and how to stop them when they occur.

This runner has a relatively lower baseline and generally stays around 80 mg/dL throughout the day (see Figure 2.3). He had a meal of a sandwich with chips and a sugary soft drink at noon, which took his glucose level from 80 to 120 mg/dL and then dropped it down to 65 mg/dL about an hour later. This is an example of a reactive hypoglycemic crash. This occurs when the athlete ingests carbs too quickly. The pancreas releases insulin pulling the glucose out of the bloodstream, but since the insulin secretion is high, it results in dropping glucose levels

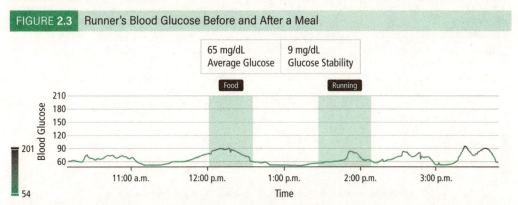

FIGURE 2.3   Runner's Blood Glucose Before and After a Meal

The timing of your meal before a workout can have a profound impact on your workout. Here a runner has a high-carb meal that causes their glucose to go up and then crash down, resulting in hypoglycemia before the start of their running workout.

below the baseline. The pancreas really has no idea how much insulin to release, well, not *no idea*, but it's not exactly certain after each meal! Moreover, it doesn't know that you need to start the workout. Therefore, after the meal and before the workout, this runner felt like he was low in blood glucose (known as "bonking" by endurance athletes), low in energy, and needed something to help bring up the glucose levels before his workout. In this case, the athlete "created" the bonk. By reducing the number of carbs, and eating healthier proteins and monounsaturated fats, he could have prevented this bonk before his workout, which he suffered just because of improper fueling.

In these two relatively uncomplicated examples, we see how timing and the volume of food intake can really make a difference between a good workout and a poor one. Now let's look at a more complicated one where Bobby Julich, a former professional cyclist who won the silver medal in the 2004 Olympics and placed third in the 1998 Tour De France, raced in a local gravel bicycle race as a Masters Athlete in the 50+ category. In Figure 2.4, we see the graph of Bobby's race. The dashed grey line is the wattage he produced, the dotted green line is his heart rate, and the solid green and black line is his glucose level. Bobby primed his system with 40 grams of carbs about 10 minutes before the race started, so he would start the race at 120mg/dL and be ready for the hard effort right at the start of the race, as these gravel races start intensely. Once he was in the front group of racers, adrenalin released and caused his body to release even more glucose from its stores of glycogen, causing his glucose to go over 200mg/dL for over 40 minutes. As the glucose lowers over the next 30 minutes, Bobby takes a gel of 30 grams of carbs to boost his glucose back up. But this was a bit too much, and his body released more insulin than needed, and he experienced a mild hyporeactive

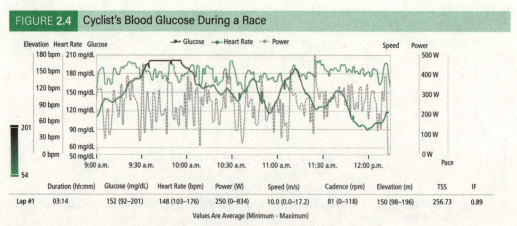

Former professional cyclist Bobby Julich races in a local masters 50+ gravel race.

glycemic crash just before 11:00 a.m. Since Bobby felt low in energy, he took in more gels, and his glucose shot up to almost 200mg/dL again, but this time the race becomes more intense and he has to respond to multiple "attacks" by the competition. He used this glucose that he just ingested in pushing harder to beat his competition, causing it to go back down again. Around 11:45 a.m., the pace eased off and his glucose swung back up, this time because the intensity of the race had lowered but also because his body was still releasing a maximum amount of glucose from the stores of glycogen in the muscles. In the last 30 minutes, his glucose dropped significantly and he needed to have another gel in order to prevent from being hypoglycemic in the final minutes of the race. As you can see, it's quite difficult for someone to time their glucose intake with the unknown intensity of a gravel bicycle race, even for someone that has had a very successful and long career as a professional.

Our next example is a pure and spicy roller coaster for a day! See Figure 2.5. This athlete started out with a big glucose spike for breakfast at 8:00 a.m., which came down at the start of the ride, and he spent the rest of the day experiencing blood glucose highs and lows. This is what you're trying to prevent! This is stressful for the body but will also give you very inconsistent feelings and energy levels throughout the ride. You'll experience high energy as the glucose increases but lower energy, and bonking, as it drops. Think of it as a struggle for the body: it continuously tries to bring your glucose to baseline or "homeostasis." Homeostasis is the condition in which your body maintains for optimal function. This is the toughest scenario to manage during a ride and especially during a race. We'll see another example of this in Chapter 6. After each drop in glucose, the athlete ate more carbs causing a peak of glucose. His pancreas overreacted releasing too much insulin, driving the glucose levels down and causing the athlete to eat another high-carb, high-glycemic food to raise his glucose and

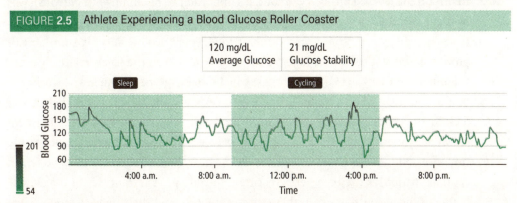

This athlete started out with a big glucose spike at breakfast, which came down at the start of the ride, followed by blood glucose highs and lows.

energy levels. This culminated in a peak after five hours of riding, as the group he was riding with decided to race the final hour home. He drank a Red Bull and ate a candy bar just before this section and hoped that it would be enough to get him to the finish without a serious hypoglycemic crash. Once you're on the "roller coaster," it's not only tough to get off, but you have to accept your fate and just keep pounding carbs to the finish and hope you've enough in your pockets to make it to the finish line. In this case, he did make it, but just barely, as you can see by the big crash at 4:00 p.m. Fortunately, it was an easy 15-minute journey home followed by a recovery shake and meal. After the activity, observe how his glucose levels stabilize and maintain equilibrium. This is a great example of what to prevent in a race or hard training ride. In this case, the athlete started off with a poor breakfast selection and then ate simple, high-glycemic carbs the entire day, instead of choosing lower-glycemic, complex carbs with some proteins and fats, which could have made a big difference.

Four different athletes, with different timings, foods, and training, results in four different outcomes. There is no "one-size-fits-all" in blood glucose. To determine the optimal timing for your training and competition, you'll have to do some experimentation to learn what works for your body. There are some important guidelines that you should consider in timing your ingestion of carbs:

1. **Prime the system**: For an intense workout or competition, you should "prime" the system, by intaking glucose 10 to 15 minutes before the beginning of your effort. This works best if you're going to be "full gas" from the start of the workout or competition, and shortcuts the time it would normally take for your body to respond and dump glucose from the liver into the bloodstream. This can give you an advantage right from the start.

2. **Maintain the levels**: During a workout, it's important to maintain your glucose levels by regularly intaking glucose and proteins, so that you don't just "spike" your glucose. If you're using simple sugars in a drink or food, you'll need to include some sort of protein and/or fat to mute a blood glucose spike and keep the levels relatively even. It's important that you make sure to test which product (type and quantity) works the best in your case (in terms of glucose time-to-response and the max peak) before you lock in the training and/or competition protocol. Another tip that helps is to sip slowly but often, rather than taking a gel in one go. This can create a more stable response. One athlete I have coached loves the little gummy chews as their preferred sports nutrition, as they can perfectly titrate the dosage. They put two of the chews/blocks in their mouth, suck on them for five minutes and then chew them up. They watch their glucose levels and if they stay the same after five more minutes, they'll

repeat with two more chews/blocks and continue this way until they start moving the trending arrow upward. This is a much better way to maintain your level instead of stuffing eight of them in your mouth at once, and creating a big spike and possible hypo crash.

3. **Sometimes you need a spike**! There are many times during your training and/or competition that you'll need sugar and need it now! This generally happens when you're low and on the verge of hypoglycemia (bonking).

4. **Eating too early can be bad**: Traditionally, athletes have been told to eat three hours before their event. While having a solid meal three hours before the event or training allows you to digest the foods more completely, if you don't supplement with other foods within the hour before your effort, you could have low glucose levels at the start. It's fine to eat three hours before your event or training (giving your body the time to get back to homeostasis). Just know that the hour before, you'll want to make sure you watch your CGM and see how your glucose is doing so you can ingest more food if needed.

5. **Avoid the roller coaster**! It's important to avoid the blood glucose roller coaster. This results in poor workouts and events, is stressful on your body, and isn't great for your mood. You can prevent this by avoiding simple, high-glycemic carbs especially before and during the initial part of your workout or event. More complex, low-glycemic carbs are better in the beginning and throughout your workout to avoid this nasty situation.

6. **Once on the roller coaster, accept it**: If you find yourself on the blood glucose roller coaster, you just have to keep it going. Watch your CGM carefully and when you see your blood glucose coming down more than 30 mg/dL from its peak, you need to start ingesting more carbs to prevent the crash at the bottom. You can carefully arrest this drop, but it takes practice and discipline. I've found that most athletes find this difficult to do, especially once the competition has started.

Sequencing of Food Intake

How does the order of the food that you intake impact your glucose levels? Does this matter during training or competition, or in life for that matter? Can you make a profound change in your body's response just by reordering your food intake?

What I mean by food sequencing is that the order in which you ingest your food matters. Most of us sit down at the table with a plate of food and move from one food to the other, eating whichever food next that takes our fancy. We never think about the order of carbs, proteins, and fats on our plate, and many times the foods we eat have all three ingredients in them. However, by "stacking" your food correctly, you can reduce the blood glucose rise and maintain a longer and more moderate amount of blood glucose. This is a simple yet revolutionary way to eat your meals, which does take a little discipline but no extra energy.

Start with your salad first, eat it completely. Heck, you might do this anyway! Maybe this is why salad is always served first at restaurants. When you eat salad, use only olive oil and vinegar as the dressing. This avoids the nasty sugars that are used in most commercial dressings, and avoids seed oils, which are not great for you (more on that in Chapter 8). The vinegar in the dressing contains acetic acid. While it's not entirely clear what mechanism causes your glucose to lower after ingesting vinegar, there are some scientific theories.

The acetic acid in vinegar increases the rate at which glucose uptake occurs in the muscles, most likely from an improvement in insulin action in skeletal muscle. Vinegar also has been proven to enhance glycogen repletion in animal studies.[23] This combination can reduce the glucose rise that you might see without including vinegar first. It's also thought that vinegar can reduce gastric emptying. In a study, admittedly small, of 10 healthy, regular weight people, scientists observed that indeed, vinegar reduced both blood glucose levels and insulin concentrations after a high-starch meal. They wrote: "The mechanism is probably a delayed gastric emptying rate."[24] Another interesting study done on rats using balsamic vinegar found that it improves the function of beta cells in the pancreas, and those beta cells are the ones that secrete insulin in response to the presence of glucose in the blood.[25] Yet another study found a third possible mechanism in which vinegar may interfere with disaccharidases, which are enzymes in the small intestine that break down carbohydrates. This will reduce the absorption of carbohydrates and slow down the glucose emptying into the bloodstream.[26]

With the food stacking method in mind, now let's stack your veggies on top of the salad. Eat all of your vegetables next. Don't have a bite of carbs or protein while eating your vegetables, eat all your vegetables completely. By adding in additional fiber, any carbohydrates coming later will be even more slowly absorbed. After your vegetables, eat all your protein. Again, eat all the protein, whether that is tofu or steak, eat it all now. Finally, eat your carbs. (Isn't it interesting that tradition is that we always have our sweets or dessert last!) This is the top of the food stack and will be digested later and more slowly as your body has to work through the fiber and proteins first, with the carbs coming in more slowly. The impact this has on your blood glucose is profound! Try eating the same dinner two days in a row and looking at your CGM data to see the differences. When you food stack, the spike will be much, much lower and you'll have a longer supply of blood glucose in your system that is more stable. In Figure 2.6, we see a dinner that has been eaten using the food stacking method, and in Figure 2.7, we see the exact same meal not stacked.

Food stacking is good for training and competition purposes, as it is for life. By making a simple yet revolutionary change to the order of how you eat foods, you can improve your

CHAPTER 2: How Foods Impact Your Glucose and Performance   29

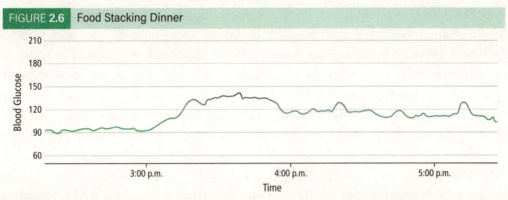

By eating your foods in a certain order, you can minimize your glucose response. "Food Stacking" can make a real difference.

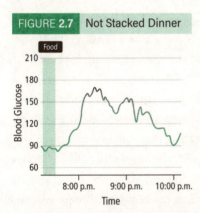

The same meal eaten not using the stacking method results in a much higher glucose level and steeper decline.

energy for your workouts and your events. In your daily life, this will also reduce your average daily blood glucose, the peaks of your spikes, and the stress on your pancreas. The change can be so great that I recommend it for everyone, not just athletes.

BLOOD GLUCOSE HACKS

There are numerous ways that you can reduce your blood glucose spike, both the peak of it and the duration of the rise. Why would you want to do this though? For those that might already be in the prediabetic range using the hemoglobin A1C (HbA1c) measure from 5.7 to 6.4, it's important to significantly reduce your blood glucose spikes and improve your insulin sensitivity. Yes, it's reversible and by changing lifestyle and habits around food and exercise, you can do a lot to improve your HbA1c. If you're below 5.7, in the normal range, then it's also important to reduce your spikes, because you don't want to become prediabetic in the future and want to maintain a more stable level of blood glucose. Constantly raising your blood glucose up and down on the "roller coaster," affects your energy level, mood, and ability to maintain focus.

Let's also consider your daily average blood glucose number. Even if you've a very normal and healthy glucose/insulin response to high-glycemic foods, constantly spiking your glucose levels to 180–200 mg/dL and over will absolutely raise your daily average blood glucose and HbA1c. For example, if you're cruising along at 90 mg/dL, then have a meal that is predominately high glycemic and your blood glucose rises to 180 mg/dL within 30 minutes, and then drops back down to 90 mg/dL at 75 minutes after your meal, your average blood glucose might be 135 mg/dL for that entire 75 minutes. Conversely, if you ensure that you eat a low-glycemic meal and your blood glucose rises to 120 mg/dL and back down to 90 mg/dL again, your average might be 100 mg/dL over the 75 minutes. Raising your blood glucose to a high level, even if you've very normal and good insulin sensitivity, will increase your daily average glucose. This might not matter for an occasional meal but if you do this every day for a lifetime, it could cause you to become a type 2 diabetic later in life (alongside other risk factors).

Conversely, I want to encourage you to not obsess about keeping your glucose low all the time. Repeat after me: "Keto (and the carnivore diet) is *not* the answer. Keto is *not* the answer. Keto is *not* the answer." Many of you'll start with your CGM and see all those blood glucose spikes as you eat your normal diet that you've been eating all your life. Then you'll experiment with just eating protein and fats, and find that those spikes go away. Yes, they go away because you're not ingesting any carbohydrates, so of course your blood glucose is not going to rise. However, by increasing your protein (animal and vegan) and your fats, especially saturated fat, you're very likely to be causing long-term trouble (more on this later). As an athlete working to improve, presumably you'll be doing some high intensity exercise, and these require carbohydrates! To do those efforts over 80% of your threshold heart rate, you'll need carbs and stored glycogen in the muscles and liver. Yes, there are athletes out there that run on pure protein and fats, but they're limited to very low-intensity exercises. Again, the answer is not keto. You're not going to improve your performance by going keto. You do need carbs, and blood glucose spikes are normal. Let's just make sure that we eat foods that are reducing those peaks and maintaining a more stable supply of energy.

Hacks to Reduce Glucose Spikes

Apple cider vinegar. This is a well-known hack that you can ingest 30 minutes before you eat a high-carbohydrate meal. Most studies have all focused around using two tablespoons (10 mL) of apple cider vinegar (ACV) mixed with three to four ounces of water 30 minutes before your meal. This absolutely works, as mentioned earlier in this chapter under the section "Sequencing of Food Intake." There are many studies to back up this phenomenon and I encourage you to dig deeper into the referenced studies earlier in this chapter.

Lemon/lime juice. Squeeze some lemon/lime slices into your water at mealtimes. These also contain citric acid and will work similarly to how the acetic acid in ACV works to help reduce your spikes. This is another great reason to drink water with your meals.

Ketone esters. Ketone esters (KEs) like what is made by the industry standard company, deltaG®, can reduce your blood glucose spikes and your steady-state blood glucose too. One study found that by ingesting a KE drink 30 minutes before an oral glucose tolerance test, reduced circulating glucose by 11% in adults with obesity, 15% in young, healthy participants and improved glycemic response by 17%. "A reduction in steady-state glucose by 10% was observed by both nonobese and obese adults. The mechanisms underlying the glucose-lowering effects of KE are not entirely clear. The small, yet immediate, increase in insulin secretion after KE ingestion may be sufficient to inhibit hepatic glucose production."[27]

Alcohol. While I do *not* recommend this to help mute your blood glucose spikes and reduce the circulating blood glucose in your bloodstream, it does work. When the impact of alcohol was studied on healthy, lean individuals, it was found that a relatively small amount of alcohol (about one and a half drinks) consumed an hour before a high-carb meal can reduce post-meal glucose levels and even lower insulin levels, as compared to eating the same meal without alcohol.[28] It's a range that depends on the person, as some reduced their glucose by 16% whereas others reduced it by 37%.

So why is this happening? First off, alcohol inhibits the production of new glucose in the liver through the gluconeogenesis process, which can lead to lower circulating blood glucose levels. Secondly, light to moderate alcohol consumption can potentially result in a short-term increase in insulin sensitivity,[29] which would cause a better uptake of glucose from your meal and enhanced sugar uptake from your meal into the cells. The effects of alcohol are somewhat controversial and based on my own observation of athletes using a CGM, it appears to depend highly on the person. The effects of alcohol highly impact some and others not as much, in terms of inebriation and glucose levels. Again, this is *not* a recommended way to reduce your blood glucose and certainly won't help improve your athletic performance. Drinking any amount of alcohol is known to be detrimental to your body and performance.[30]

CHAPTER 3

The Steps to Using Your CGM

WHAT IS YOUR OPTIMAL GLUCOSE LEVEL for performance? How does it change at different intensities? What about right before your workout or competition? Where should you maintain your glucose level during your event? What are important metrics to watch out for during your workout?

I mentioned this at the end of Chapter 1, but 1 want to reiterate it here because it's so important. Keep this in the back of your head as you read this book: the effects of your food on glucose levels are dependent on many factors, including mood, the last time you ate, how long you've been fasting (overnight for example), and your training status. Your glucose level could be vastly different at the end of a three-week training block than it will be after one week of rest. Glucose levels can also be influenced by your sleep quality and any stress you are experiencing outside of your exercise life.

STEP 1: GATHER DATA

When you first apply your continuous glucose monitor (CGM), your goal is to gather data and observe your individual trends. You might want to change your diet every time you see your glucose levels spike, but you need to resist this temptation. Gather at least two weeks of data on your normal diet. Whatever you're eating now is your normal diet. After you've established that norm, then you can start making changes as you go along. With your new CGM, you'll want to track all meals and snacks, exercise, and sleep to make sure you capture all glucose metrics for these. You'll do this is by creating an "event" (different apps call it different things, but we'll call them events for the purpose of this book). When tracking your meals, you should create a new event when you start eating a meal, and end the event *after* there has been a blood glucose spike and it comes back down to your equilibrium point or normal average blood glucose. This way the event captures before the meal, the response of the blood glucose after the meal and when it comes back down at the end of the meal to your norm. This is important. See Figure 3.0.

33

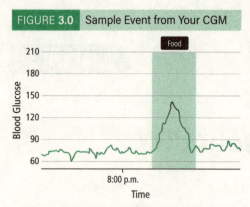

Be sure to create a range around your entire glucose spike to ensure you have the correct average glucose value for it.

You'll do the same for your sleep, when you wake up in the morning. Open your CGM app and mark the time you went to sleep, which is usually characterized by a sudden drop in blood glucose (unless of course you ate a big bowl of ice cream and chocolate sauce before bed, then it will continue to go up during your sleep!) and encompass your full sleep period to when you wake in the morning and get out of bed.

....

Note: If you shower in the morning, then you'll see a "fake" spike (also called an "artifact" of the sensor) because of the sharp temperature swing of the water. This is not a real change in your blood glucose, but a result of the temperature sensor inside the CGM measuring incorrectly because of the sudden change in temperature. This can also occur if you go into a sauna or if you go from a warm home into the cold outdoors.

....

STEP 2: LEARN YOUR BASELINE

The first thing you should do when you get your CGM applied is to learn your average daily glucose levels and observe what is getting you out of that 70–140 milligrams per deciliter (mg/dL) zone. This is done simply by wearing the CGM and observing what your "normal," or basal, levels are when your body is in glucose homeostasis. Your body wants to maintain your glucose levels in a narrow window, so it's constantly striving to get back to that stable level. You find yours by looking at the average glucose after you've eaten, and then allowing the glucose levels to rise and come back down and stabilize. For example, let's say that your glucose is trucking along at a pre-meal baseline of 85 mg/dL. You eat a nice healthy meal of vegetables and fruits with a little plant-based protein in there and observe that your glucose increases to 124 mg/dL 30 minutes after you finish your meal. Within 90 minutes after your meal, it stabilizes at 90–95 mg/dL (close to your pre-meal baseline) and stays there for the next three hours. In these circumstances, your daily baseline blood glucose level would be 90–95 mg/dL. (A true scientific baseline is a morning, fasted baseline.) What's a normal baseline? Again, there is no normal as everyone is different, but according to the latest science:[31]

Normal range: 4–6 millimoles per liter (mmol/L) or 72–108 mg/dL.

Lab-Based Blood Glucose Testing

Lab-based testing is required for the appropriate diagnosis of diabetes mellitus.

Prediabetes

Impaired fasting glucose range: 5.7–6.4 mmol/L or 100–125 mg/dL.

Impaired oral glucose tolerance test range at two hours post-75 g oral glucose ingestion: 7.8–11.0 mmol/L or 140–199 mg/dL.

A recent study with 12,504 active healthy participants revealed "small differences between genders in overall 24-hour glycemia, with women having slightly lower 24-hour mean glucose levels as well as lower glucose levels in response to meals and sleep than men."[32] See Figure 3.1. So, what are you striving to achieve and keep? If you're not prediabetic, your glucose level should be less than 100 mg/dL as a daily average.

STEP 3: UNDERSTAND YOUR RESPONSES

Now you get to have some fun and do some experiments! Yay! This is very exciting because you get to eat all kinds of foods and see what happens to your glucose levels. The key to these experiments is to make sure you accurately record and learn from them. In Appendix A, we've provided a place for you to write down your foods, your beginning, peak, and average glucose numbers, and the length of time it took to return to pre-meal baseline. You may wish to note any unusual

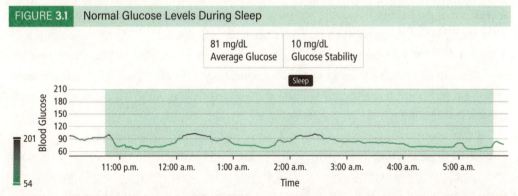

FIGURE 3.1 Normal Glucose Levels During Sleep

You want your glucose levels to be under 100 mg/dL on average for your entire day, including the period when you are sleeping.

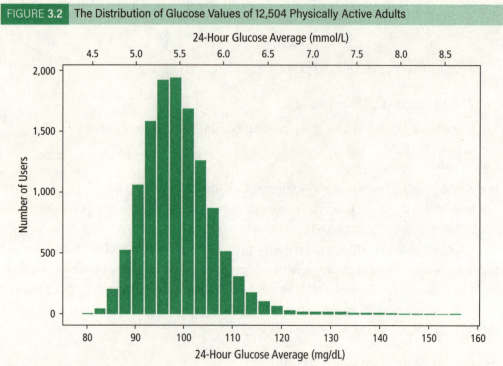

FIGURE 3.2 The Distribution of Glucose Values of 12,504 Physically Active Adults

A population's 24-hour glucose average.

factors that might have impacted the measurement positively or negatively, and your emotional state (feeling good, having negative thoughts, and your level of stress and/or fatigue, etc.).

Where to start? As an "N=1" or the test subject. You'll need to be willing to give these a try so that you can learn your individual responses. Before we go any farther, repeat after me: It's not about keto, it's not about keto, it's *not* about keto. I know I've mentioned this before and I'll mention it again later in this book, but there can be a strong temptation to go all protein/fat after seeing blood glucose spikes. Consider the latest science. In a study of 12,504 physically active adults, 85% had an average daily glucose between 90 and 110 mg/dL. Note that this doesn't mean they don't leave this range, this is just their daily average. In fact, you can see in Figure 3.2, as a population, there is a fluctuation across the day. Given the size of the sample, this is a truly strong signal that is convincing.[33]

Please ensure that you read Chapter 8 about using a CGM for health to learn why it's so important to keep eating healthy carbs (Go Veggies, Go Legumes, Go Grains!) and to find out about the "fat" causation theory of type 2 diabetes. The next thing to keep in mind is that there are many variables that will impact your glucose response. Some of these are: your gender, age, and fitness level; the length, type and intensity of your workouts; your training freshness or fatigue; the amount and quality of sleep; your alcohol consumption; your gut microbiome; any macro diet you're on, like vegan or paleo, etc.; your prediabetic symptoms; and more. You can alter your responses with some changes in health, including weight loss and improvements in eating. So you could have a particular response at the beginning of this journey, but through improved eating habits, a change in diet and better sleep, you might need to completely re-read this section a year from now to understand the "new" you. This is just one reason why learning how to use your CGM for performance can be challenging. On a smaller scale, you might find that "X" food gives you a "Y" response on Monday, but on Friday, "X" food gives you a "Z" response. The most important takeaways in this section are that you're learning *your* basic responses to a few basic tests that can be repeated.

Test #1: The Roller Coaster

Your first test will be to deliberately create high glucose levels throughout the day. This is to learn the extreme (I hope it's extreme to you and not the norm!) of a real hyperglycemia spike and then a hypoglycemia low. This should be done on a rest day from training and competition, so that exercise doesn't influence the results and you don't end up ruining a critical training day. (Reminder: the results would be different if this was made on a training day.) For this test it's important to allow sufficient time, roughly 90 minutes, depending on the meal composition, between meals and snacks to allow your glucose levels to return to the basal amount and see if you're going to have any excessive drops in glucose levels at the bottom of the "roller coaster." Once you feel like you've hit bottom, pre-meal baseline or even lower, then have your next snack or meal and go back to the top of the roller coaster again. *Disclaimer: this is only for the purpose of testing and shouldn't be done on a regular basis!*

As with any experimentation on yourself, be careful and stop the experiment if you begin to have adverse medical effects. I also recommend that you do *not* do this if you're a type 1 or 2 diabetic, you've prediabetes, or if you have any chronic metabolic issue, as this will really put a load on your insulin supply and production. Just be careful people! Remember to create events around all your meals, and your sleep the night before and the night after. That way you can learn what blood glucose spikes really are and how long it takes for your body to rid itself of excessive glucose. One thing to also keep in mind when doing this experiment is that your glucose response won't be the same as if you had a sugary soft drink at lunch during your "normal" day. You're really stressing your body to the limits, and it's a very good test to see how you respond, but it's just not the same as a single sugary serving of something on a regular day.

These are options, so treat them as such. You're not meant to eat everything on the list below and you're not limited to just these foods.

Breakfast:
- Quick oats from a package with honey drizzled on top and a glass of orange juice or coffee with sugar
- Three or four doughnuts and coffee with sugar
- Toasted plain or cinnamon raisin bagel with cinnamon sugar and melted butter
- Danish or other pastries with jelly in the middle and coffee with sugar
- Fruit loops or other sugary breakfast cereal and sweetened oat milk

Mid-morning snack:
- Candy bar
- Rice cakes
- Snack bag of potato chips
- Sugary energy drink

Lunch:
- Jif, or equivalent, peanut butter and jelly sandwich on white or wheat bread
- Chick-fil-A chicken sandwich or equivalent sandwich and fries (make sure to eat the bun!)
- Rice and bean burrito and tortilla chips

Mid-afternoon snack:
- Four fig bars
- Two Pop-Tarts
- Candy bar
- Six chocolate chip cookies
- Drink a soda as well just for fun!

Dinner:
- Pasta with red sauce (make sure it contains sugar in the ingredient label)
- White rice, rolls, mac and cheese, and a Coke
- Asian noodles with veggies and protein
- Three or four slices of pepperoni or your favorite pizza

Dessert:
- Ice cream
- Cake with chocolate sauce
- Marshmallow s'mores

Reminder: these are options! You are not meant to eat the whole list under each meal.

What's the goal? The goal is to learn how high your glucose levels will go, to establish a correlation between these high-glycemic foods and other foods you might eat. Secondly, you want to see how quickly your glucose levels drop after each meal and how far it drops. A normal glucose response to a high-glycemic food is made of a glucose curve that rises to its peak in approximately 30 minutes (more or less) and comes back to baseline within 90 minutes. If it drops quickly from your peak glucose, then it's likely you've no issues with prediabetes or diabetes. If it stays high for a much longer period and doesn't come down, then it's *possible* you *might* have some of the warning signs of prediabetes. When your glucose levels come down and drop below the level it was before the meal, then you've induced a reactive hypoglycemic crash or a low blood sugar crash and you'll want to observe your feelings. Are you having negative feelings or bad thoughts when your glucose is low? Are you feeling good and have positive happy thoughts when it's high? Are you neutral and not feeling good or bad? When are you sleepy, yawning, and tired? What was your average glucose for the day? For the night? How was your workout? Can you imagine doing this every day?

Test #2: Let's Go Keto

I suggest that the very next day, you go completely the opposite way and see how this feels. What does that mean? No carbs at all. Only eat proteins and fats for all your meals and snacks. Eliminate all carbs from your diet for at least 15 hours. Observe your glucose levels and compare this to the previous day. Make sure you eliminate all sugars and carbs, even the sweetener in your coffee.

What's the goal? To learn what happens when you only eat protein and fats, and to see how your blood glucose responds to the lack of sugar/carbs; and to learn how this makes you feel. Did you get any headaches? Did you feel energized? How was your workout? Can you imagine eating this way every day?

It's possible you might need to do two days of keto to really eliminate the excess glucose from your body and see how this feels.

Test #3: The Sports Gel Test

Give yourself a few days of rest after the two previous tests, find your baseline again and enjoy your normal diet. After you feel like you're seeing normal responses again, then the next morning after you wake up, before your coffee, before your breakfast, check out your CGM, note the number and then take three sports gels that are fast-acting high-glycemic glucose/fructose gels.

TABLE 3.0 Are You a Fast, Medium, or Slow Responder?

Type of response	Fast	Medium	Slow
Length of time from baseline to peak and back to baseline.	Less than 60 minutes	61–90 minutes	91 minutes+*
Percentage rise of blood glucose peak from baseline.	250%+	150–250%	Less than 150%
Drop from baseline to post-baseline (subtract post-baseline number from pre-meal number). A hypoglycemic "trough." This indicates if you had a hypo crash or not.	20–40 mg/dL	10–20 mg/dL	0–10 mg/dL
Rise or fall of blood glucose one hour after sports gel. How much did your blood glucose change at the one-hour point?	0–15 mg/dL	16–50 mg/dL	51+ mg/dL
Rise or fall of blood glucose two hours after sports gel. How much did your blood glucose change at the two-hour point?	0–15 mg/dL	16–30 mg/dL	31+ mg/dL

Prediabetics will most likely have an even longer time from the baseline to peak and back to baseline. This doesn't mean that they're slow responders, but have some level of insulin resistance. Impaired glucose tolerance (prediabetes) is diagnosed by measuring a person's blood glucose two hours after a drink with 75 g glucose in it. If a person's glucose is 7.8 mmol/L (140 mg/dL) or above two hours after the drink, this is impaired glucose tolerance.

It's important that you stay relatively inactive for one to two hours, because if you're active afterward, this will reduce your circulating glucose and negate the test.

Do this test twice. Wait two days and do it again, so you can ensure that your first result was the correct and normal response. It's important to eat what you would eat the night before an event or hard workout. If you have a huge meal the night before at 9:00 p.m., and then stay up till 11:00 p.m., then get up at 6:00 a.m. and eat your gels, your numbers will be vastly different than what you would see if you had a salad and went to bed at 9:00 p.m. So it's important to minimize the variables here the day and night before, so that both of the sports gel tests can be compared to each other. Note: This is not fun. You're breaking a fast and then you're going on a glucose "ride."

What's the goal? To categorize yourself as a fast, medium or slow responder to a pure sugar sports gel (see Table 3.0).[34] This will help you to determine optimal timing for a pre-workout or competition drink, gel, or meal. It's important to understand how quickly you clear glucose out of your blood. Those who are fast responders could easily time their sports nutrition too far out from an effort and have a big crash at the start of a competition. Those who are slower responders don't need to worry as much about timing their pre-competition nutrition too far out but need to be concerned with making sure it's not too close to the event, as then they might not have their blood glucose up high enough to perform well. These are general guidelines, and the numbers below assume that you are neither a type 1 or type 2 diabetic, nor prediabetic. It's always good to recheck your time-to-response in a race-specific situation (for example, prior to the race-specific workout). You should also consider the hormonal response that a competition will create; it represents an important stress for the body and the glucose response might be enhanced by adrenalin (for example). There is a difference between male and female glucose levels and these need to be taken into consideration. Females have slightly lower average glucose values than males in all respects: food, exercise, sleep, and as a daily average.[35] Finally, some people just have low glucose levels and that's their norm.[36] It's not entirely clear why this occurs, and more research is needed with this in mind.

Now, color in where you fit with the grid above and see if you're predominantly one or the other. It's quite possible you fit into two categories.

What are you going to do with this newfound information? This will help you with the timing of your sports nutrition, and your workouts and events. The fast responders will need to be much more careful about ingesting any high-glycemic foods more than an hour out from their workout or competition. They'll need to maintain a more constant supply of complex carbs in smaller doses and throughout the two hours leading up to their effort. These athletes will need to be very careful with ingesting simple sugars too far out from the start of their workout or an event. Conversely, they can have some simple sugars within 10 minutes of their event and start it with a moderate/high level of blood glucose so they're ready to go hard from the start. (Read more about this in Chapter 5.) If you're a fast responder and eat too early before your effort, you risk starting that effort after your blood glucose has spiked and dropped, and possibly dropped into the hypoglycemic trough that can occur after your meal/sports nutrition. See Figure 3.3. Fast responders need to be very careful in the timing of their sports nutrition. The type of carbs that you ingest is very important to recognize, as a sucrose (simple sugar) sports drink could have a vastly different response than a maltodextrin sports drink, than a glucose/fructose blend sports drink. A slow-digesting sports drink with starch as its main source of carbohydrates, like in the UCAN® sports drink, will definitely do its job and lower your response and peak, so keep this in mind.

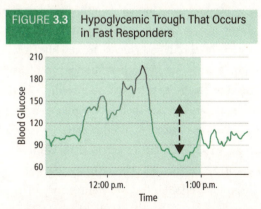

FIGURE 3.3 Hypoglycemic Trough That Occurs in Fast Responders

If you are a fast responder, you need to be careful to time your sports nutrition correctly.

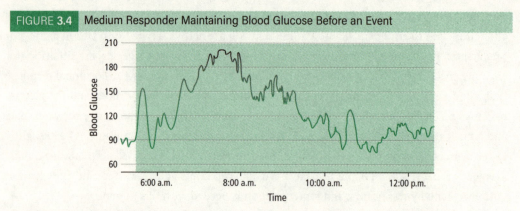

FIGURE 3.4 Medium Responder Maintaining Blood Glucose Before an Event

A medium responder maintains glucose levels longer but still needs to optimize sports nutrition timing.

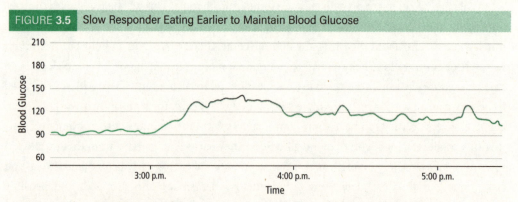

FIGURE 3.5 Slow Responder Eating Earlier to Maintain Blood Glucose

A slow responder needs simple carbs before an event in order to raise levels for a peak performance.

Medium responders also need to be concerned with timing and what they eat before an event, but not as much. See Figure 3.4. These athletes can eat a little earlier and still maintain a good level of blood glucose for a while. It will still be important to ingest both complex and simple carbs, but medium responders can easily sustain energy levels for a longer time. They'll need to ensure that they've some simple sugars before their event, at least 20 to 30 minutes before, to make sure their blood glucose rises enough for the start of the event.

Slower responders need even more time before an event to eat and raise their blood glucose, so should plan to eat healthy complex and simple carbs around two hours out from event. See Figure 3.5. This way, by the start of the workout or event, their blood glucose has risen high enough to give them plenty of energy. These athletes need to have a little more simple carbohydrates than the high and medium responding athletes, to raise their blood glucose at all. Sometimes, they've trouble raising their blood glucose, so it might be the case that they could ingest double the amount of simple carbohydrates than a fast responder might need. I suggest if you're in this category, eating a well-balanced and easy-to-digest meal two hours out from your event, then having 40 g of carbs about 15 to 20 minutes before your workout or event, will allow you to raise your blood glucose so that at the start of the effort you'll be primed and ready to go.

Remember to keep in mind that glucose response depends on your training state, stress absence/presence, hormonal response, sleeping quality, amount of carbs in your previous meal, etc.

Test #4: The Whole Foods, Plant-Based Test

This is a great test as it will show you how your blood glucose might change if you've a purely plant-based meal. Now, when you make this meal, you need to make sure there are no *oils* in the meal and you don't use any when cooking. Oils will dramatically change the results of this test, so it's important to steer clear of them.

I suggest making a meal that contains at least five different vegetables (steamed, sauteed, or baked), one serving of legumes (beans), one serving of complex carb (brown rice, tempeh, or quinoa), and one fruit of your choice.

What's the goal? In this test, you want to understand just how eating plants cooked without oils impact your blood glucose. How much did it rise? Did it rise at all? Was it satisfying for you, or did it leave you wanting more? If you're left wanting more, then have extra servings but don't eat animal proteins. In this test, it's also important to see how you feel after three hours, so please note your energy levels and blood glucose number at three hours for this test. If your blood glucose has dropped slowly or more rapidly, then you'll have a better idea of how to fuel if you eat this kind of meal throughout your day. If your blood glucose drops rapidly and you become hypoglycemic, then you'll want to add in some plant-based protein the next time, like tofu, soybeans, legumes, pea protein, and soy crumbles. If your blood glucose drops slowly over a longer period, this means that your plant-based meal reacted well with your body as is and there's no need for additional plant-based proteins. More and more athletes are learning that plant-based meals are the key to longevity, and that they can get enough nutrients with the right balance of foods.

STEP 4: DEFINE YOUR GLUCOSE PERFORMANCE ZONES

Yay! More testing! Mood, movement, and nutrition are the three main drivers of your blood glucose values, so it's important to understand how movement plays into this and define your optimal glucose performance zone (GPZ). Your GPZ is a concept to help you derive feedback from your CGM. Specifically, it's defined as the range of glucose where you perform and feel best. This may be a broad or narrow range, and it may differ between sports and intensities. It should be noted that glucose may not change a great deal from baseline when undertaking low-intensity steady-state activity but will primarily be driven up by intensity and carbohydrate intake.

The GPZ should not be seen as an ideal area for your glucose to be during all exercise. It is merely a concept to help you better evaluate your fueling during activity; it's a visual rather than physiological concept.

The key here is basically repeating Step 1: Gather Data (see page 33) to a point in which you feel comfortable that you know at what range of blood glucose you feel strong during your workouts and competitions. This might be a very simple thing that you figure out within a month (I believe you need at least a month of data before you can establish your GPZ) or you might need three months of various workouts and competitions.

I have researched GPZs for over two years with over 50 athletes, in different sports, and with different ages, diets, and fitness levels—from beginner recreational to professional level. What I've found is that the ranges can vary across all athletes. This can even fluctuate week-to-week depending on the volume and intensity of your training. For example, I've worked with a whole-foods, plant-based cyclist that performs optimally within a range of 80 to 110 mg/dL. I've worked with professional cyclists that ride at their best from 140 to 200 mg/dL. I've worked with bodybuilders that have their best lifts and workouts in a tight range from 90 to 110 mg/dL. I've observed triathletes that have a GPZ from 120 to 150 mg/dL at the beginning of a new phase of training (after a rest week), go to a GPZ of 75 to 90 mg/dL in the third week of their build cycle, where they're highly fatigued and pushing to the limits. I, as a 50s Masters cyclist, perform best when my blood glucose is from 115 to 150 mg/dL.

What this variability means is that you'll need to recognize that you've different optimal GPZs throughout your training phases. It's important that you understand them and use them to optimize your training and competition.

Here's some observations that I've made over the past two years working with athletes:

1. If you're a fast responder from Step 3, then it's likely that your GPZs will be above 125 mg/dL and below 200 mg/dL. It's possible that you could even be above 140 mg/dL. This also means that you'll need to have access to more food and eat on a more regular basis, even every 30 minutes, while working out.
2. If you're a slow responder from Step 3, then it's likely that your GPZs will be lower; likely less than 110 mg/dL , all the way down to 75 mg/dL. I have watched elite runners run some of their fastest half and full marathons with an average of 75 mg/dL. That doesn't mean they might not have been able to go even faster at 90 mg/dL, but they created personal records at that level.

3. The more fatigued you become over a three-week build cycle of training, the lower your average GPZ will be. Your GPZ will be based on how well you fuel during training and how well you refuel after training and before your next session. So while I believe it's normal to see your GPZ drop over a three-week cycle of training, it's also not optimizing your performance. I would also argue that if you start out with a GPZ of 100 to 125 mg/dL and in the third week of training, no matter what you eat, you can't keep your blood glucose over 100 mg/dL while training, this is an indication that you've not replenished enough carbohydrates over the three weeks and that alone is contributing to fatigue.

4. Conversely, as you become more and more rested, your glycogen stores will fill, both in your liver and in your muscles, and your GPZs will rise. This means that if you have a taper/rest week before a key event or peak competition, it's likely you'll see very high blood glucose levels during your competition. This should not worry or shock you. Recognize it as normal and "scale up" your decisions. If in a normal training state you might ingest additional carbohydrates when you've dropped from 120 to 100 mg/dL, now you might ingest carbohydrates when you've dropped from 160 to 140 mg/dL.

5. If you find it difficult to push your blood glucose over 120 mg/dL no matter how much simple sugars you consume, then it's likely your GPZs are much lower and in the 75–100 mg/dL range.

6. If you find it very easy to raise your blood glucose over 150 mg/dL, then it's likely your ranges will be from 130 to 180 mg/dL.

The caveat to all of this is:

1. Every exercise intensity can have its own GPZ. You could have a specific GPZ for tennis and a completely different one for CrossFit.

2. Some people will have a very clear correlation between their training zones (heart rate, pace, or power on the bicycle) and their GPZs, but for others, there will be no clear relationship. As we continue to learn more about glucose and exercise, I'm confident we'll continue to refine the GPZs.

3. If you're not fasted, your glucose response can be highly variable, and what you eat in the meal before will impact your training.

4. There is a difference between males and females in both their glucose responses and GPZs. Females typically have a lower GPZ than males.

5. The moment you eat something in training, the glucose variability increases.

That stated, there is value in working to find your GPZs. Right now, your job is to collect more data and make sure to observe, during and post-workout, the ranges of your blood glucose levels when you were performing your best. Use these as your guideline and then make small adjustments from there as you learn more. For those of you that compete, ensure that you've at least four competitions worth of data. This will give you a wider range of data, guaranteeing you have seen different foods before, during, and after your competition, along with understanding where and when you felt the strongest.

STEP 5: BEGIN TRAINING AND USING THIS DATA TO REGULATE YOUR BLOOD GLUCOSE FOR OPTIMAL PERFORMANCE

Once you have established your GPZs, it's time to go training—the fun part! There are many things to consider with your blood glucose during training and the number one being that you maintain a stable and relatively high level of blood glucose (within your GPZ of course) throughout your workout. Whether you're playing pickleball at 6:00 a.m. before work for an hour or if you're competing in a full-distance triathlon, the longer you can keep your blood glucose up, the better your ability to perform. As an endurance athlete coach for over 28 years, I know that most athletes' poor workouts and finishing results come from a poor nutritional strategy that doesn't allow them to perform to their highest ability. Once you nail this part of your training and competing, then you can "check the box" and focus on tactics, strategy, technique, and mental toughness. While all sports demand a high level of competence and technical ability honed by thousands of hours of training, all that can be unraveled with a simple drop in blood glucose at the wrong time. I personally know one athlete that lost the Tour de France, a 21-day race, due to a drop in blood glucose for roughly 20 minutes. That's all it takes. You can be the best athlete in the world, but if you have a drop in blood glucose at the wrong time and don't have access to nutrition, your chances at winning could be over. What you're learning is: the GPZ can be different for a long slow training vs VO2 max intervals (for example). So, GPZ needs to be seen as a visual reference of your glucose levels; you can expect it to rise more and vary more during more intense workouts while a long steady workout at low intensity will likely produce a more stable response.

WHAT NEXT?

Now that you have a little background on both CGMs and how foods impact your glucose levels, let's figure out how best to use this information to enhance your sports performance. When examining performance enhancing tech, we often think of these only during the event itself, whereas a CGM has the unique ability to help you enhance your performance before, during, and after your events, so that you can perform at your best again and again. The insight you gain from your CGM will help you to plan what to eat and when, before your event, and your sports nutrition during your event. This will ensure you reach an appropriate glucose level for your sport, and maintain it. Lastly, in the post-workout process, you can use your CGM to ensure you're replenishing your glycogen stores and helping your muscle cells to repair and adapt, to be even better for your next event.

The next chapter will cover in depth how you should use your CGM, so let's get to it!

CHAPTER 4

Using a CGM for Optimal Training, Competing, and Recovery

THIS IS THE CHAPTER YOU'VE all been waiting for! How to improve your performance using your continuous glucose monitor (CGM). Whether you're just trying to improve your CrossFit workouts, your running times with friends on the local Saturday run, or you're a serious masters cyclist looking to medal at nationals or a professional athlete, you can and will improve your performance using a CGM and the techniques, not only in this chapter but in the entire book. Your CGM is a revolutionary tool to help you increase your glucose levels when you need it, keep it stable during your efforts, and help to support recovery. The curves and graphs presented in this chapter will give you a chance to compare and analyze your own data so that you can understand what is "normal," what is lacking, and when you've succeeded in your nutrition plan. I urge you to use this book as a reference to come back to over and over, so that when you see a specific response in your own body, you'll recognize it as something you have seen before. For example, the next time you have some pizza, you might see the infamous "double bump" (biphasic spike) that pizza will give you. See Figure 4.0. Pizza gives you an initial glucose spike from the simple carbs that come from the sauce, which contains sugar, and the dough, which is highly refined. These simple carbs quickly enter the bloodstream. The second glucose level bump comes about an hour to two later as the cheese, toppings and oils (high fat!) cause your gastrointestinal tract to take a longer time to digest the pizza and convert it to glucose (also a reason you may feel sleepy after eating pizza). So your glucose levels may seem fine, or may even drop low, initially, but a few hours later you see a large glucose spike as they're converted to yet more glucose.[37]

Researchers have known for years now that a glucose spike right after your workout is critical to get glucose, proteins, and nutrients into your cells for recovery. A second glucose spike roughly one to two hours later will further enhance your muscle repair and drive more nutrients into cells, further enhancing recovery so you can work out just as hard tomorrow.[38]

49

Beelen, et.al., found that: "Consuming CHO and protein during the early phases of recovery has been shown to positively affect subsequent exercise performance and could be of specific benefit for athletes involved in multiple training or competition sessions on the same or consecutive days."[39]

GLUCOSE PRIMING

Pre-event or workout fueling has been studied since the 1970s and there have been roughly over one hundred papers written on when and what to eat before your event. These studies, in general, all center around

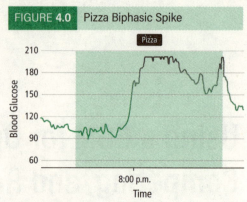

Pizza biphasic spike occurs because fats are more slowly turned into glucose and can cause the second spike two hours after eating.

feeding carbohydrates from 90 minutes to 5 minutes before your event. It's difficult to extract any meaningful advice from these, as there have been positive and negative results, sometimes negating each other. There is one study I like by Dr. Jeffrey Rothschild, et al., and it provides a good table of what to eat before an event (See Figure 4.1).[40]

There have also been many incredible books written on sports nutrition, and while I cover many topics that are also covered in these books, I'm limiting my recommendations based on the research I've done over the past two years in observing many different athletes in different sports using a CGM. It's clear to me and the athletes I've worked with that "priming" or raising your glucose before an event can be performance enhancing. There are clear issues around exactly how much and when, and this is largely because each person's glucose response is highly individual. It's important that you test and retest yourself and use the guidelines as such.

Guidelines

The first thing that you should consider, especially before a competitive event, is how to raise your glucose up to a higher level into your glucose performance zone (GPZ) so that when the event starts, you'll already be primed and ready. This is the goal in priming. You want your glucose at just the right level when the start happens. You don't want it dropping or at the bottom of a spike. You want it to be on the rise of a glucose level spike. This is not always easy to make happen as glucose levels can be impacted by many internal and external factors, so some experimentation will be important here. Good thing you have your own personal glucose lab inserted into your arm!

CHAPTER 4: Using a CGM for Optimal Training, Competing, and Recovery

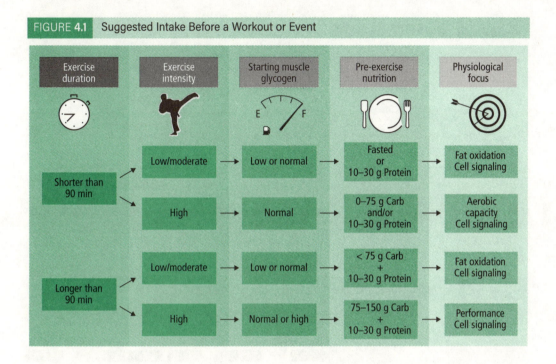

FIGURE 4.1 Suggested Intake Before a Workout or Event

Competitions that "go from the gun" demand instant high intensity, which requires a large supply of circulating glucose. However, it can take the body some time to release glucose from the stored glycogen inside the liver and muscles, so that it can enhance intensity. This lag could be as much as 10 minutes. In an event that lasts less than 10 minutes or in which the first 10 minutes are the most critical, that's too long to wait and you're certainly at a disadvantage during this lag. By priming your system, you can ensure that you start your competition or an intense training session within the optimal GPZ for you. In Figure 4.2, bodybuilder and track sprinter, Lorenzo Elder, starts a track workout without any fuels beforehand. Note how it takes about 15 minutes for his glucose to rise to meet the intense demands of a track workout and then how it drops quickly during the workout.

In Figure 4.3, we see that Lorenzo maintains much higher glucose levels for a longer period of time and, consequently, has a much better workout where he is able to do more sprints, and his speed is higher in the final sprints too. He ate two gels before this workout at the correct time (for him) and it made a huge difference. (Lorenzo's individual nutritional needs and individual CGM response that was tested previously in training.)

This works across the board for all sports, not just running on the track or weightlifting. It works for CrossFit, cycling, pickleball, etc. If you need to be at your best from the word "GO!," then you need to learn to prime yourself correctly.

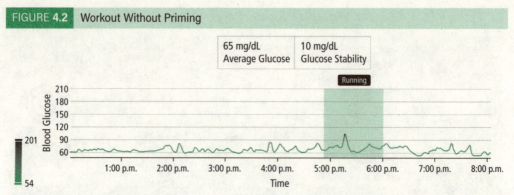

Bodybuilder and track sprinter, Lorenzo Elder, starting his workout without priming, which compromised the quality of his running.

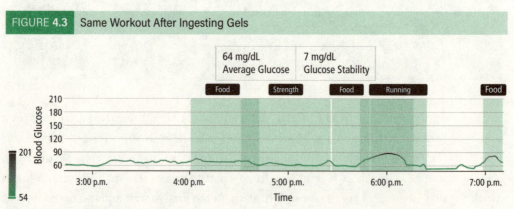

The same track workout but now starting after he ingested (two) gels, fifteen minutes before the workout.

How Should You Prime?

For fast responders. One sports gel or a 12 oz simple sugar carb drink with simple carbohydrates (remember that these could have different responses based on the types of carbs in them) and around 20–30g of carbohydrates from both glucose and fructose sources no more than 15 minutes before your event.

Fast responders also need to ensure they've some complex carbohydrates easily available to them, so when their glucose levels do come down quickly, they can preempt this drop with complex carbs coming in behind the simple carbs.

For medium responders. One sports gel or a 12 oz simple sugar carb drink with simple carbohydrates and around 20–30g of carbohydrates from both glucose and fructose sources. This absolutely must be ingested 15 minutes before, at the very latest!

For slower responders. One sports gel or a 12 oz simple sugar carb drink with simple carbohydrates and around 20–30g of carbohydrates from both glucose and fructose sources, from 45 to 30 minutes before.

A second sports gel with simple carbohydrates and around 20–30g of carbohydrates from both glucose and fructose sources or 6 oz of simple sugar carb drink 10 minutes before your event.

The slower responders will need to ingest more simple carbs, quite possibly two times what a faster responder would ingest. The caveat here is making sure that your gastrointestinal tract can tolerate it.

For everyone. You need to do some testing with different types of foods to find what works best for you and what your gastrointestinal tract tolerates the best. This can be in liquid form with a high-carb sports drink, or one to three sports gels, an easy-to-digest sports bar, three to four fig cookies, etc. There are numerous choices out there. There is some significant research showing that a blend of glucose and fructose in your gel or sports drink (honey also works) allows you to absorb more glucose across the intestinal wall.[41]

It's all about the timing!

A study by Asker Jeukendrup found that giving carbohydrates 45 minutes before an event actually hurt performance because it caused a reactive hypoglycemic crash.[42] This is exactly what we want to avoid. See Figure 4.4.

Unfortunately, this study was conducted way before commercial CGMs came on the market, and it also didn't test time periods shorter than 45 minutes or categorize athletes into different types of responders.

The key is to try a few different things. Once you've found the glucose levels response you want, stick with that product and the timing. Experimenting on yourself will be critical to ensuring that your glucose is on the rise when the start happens. I can't emphasize this enough: *timing is critical*, and you might find that none of the previous recommendations fit you. That's okay. That's why you're using them as guidelines: to help you begin to find the right timing for yourself. Be as scientific as possible with this priming protocol and you'll enhance your performance right from the word, "GO!"

Caveats and Concerns to Priming

The critical concern is that you accidentally create what is called a reactive hypoglycemic crash. This is when you have a quick rise in glucose, followed by a large insulin release and subsequent drop in glucose, so much that your glucose levels drop below your initial baseline. This, in some cases, can create the weak, dizzy, wonky feeling just before your event. Obviously, you want to avoid this.

WHAT IS A REACTIVE HYPO CRASH?

Before exercise, carbohydrate ingestion can result in high glucose levels. As soon as you start exercising, glucose levels can drop quickly because of the combined effect of high insulin levels (secreted when you ingest your priming food) and the quick uptake of glucose into the muscle cells that are needed for the creation of energy. This can easily make glucose drop very quickly and cause hypoglycemia. See Figure 4.4. This is commonly called rebound or reactive hypoglycemia.[43]
Here are some tricks for preventing a reactive hypo crash:

- If you're a fast responder, then you'll be more susceptible to this reaction. Therefore, you need to be very careful to ensure you have easy and quick access to additional complex and simple carbs before your event. This means that if you see your glucose levels dropping quickly, you can slam some more carbs instantly and prevent it.
- Ingesting complex carbs with simple carbs nearly every time you need to fuel during exercise reduces the chances of this occurring, as the complex carbs help to reduce the glucose peak and maintain glucose levels longer.
- Drink UCAN®, a sports drink proven to prevent reactive hypo crashes. UCAN® is a relatively new sports drink on the market and was created by a neurochemist whose friend's son was born with Glycogen Storage Disease, a rare genetic disorder that prevented his liver from converting glycogen to glucose. This neurochemist created a new, natural carbohydrate, called LIVSTEADY®, that not only cured his friend's son and hundreds of other kids with this disorder, but also gives the user a quick but smaller spike of glucose and then a longer, more stable release as well. This super-starch was rapidly recognized to have a great benefit to athletes and has come to be used in gels, bars, and drinks like UCAN®. It does work, and I've hundreds of data files showing workout data with glucose data, proving that it does provide the athlete with a quick spike and then a steady

glucose for longer. Sometimes too well, and slow responders might not get the spike in glucose levels that they need by using it. UCAN® is a branched cluster dextrin (HBCD), which is a type of carbohydrate derived from cornstarch. Because of its high molecular weight and low osmolality (the measure of the number of dissolved particles in the fluid), it causes faster gastric emptying and faster absorption to give you an initial glucose levels spike, which is lower than drinking a pure sucrose, glucose, etc. sports drink. HBCD also provides a sustained release of energy, keeping your glucose levels up for a longer time due to its slow breakdown in the body.

- Along with your gel or carb drink, and if your gastrointestinal tract tolerates it well, then a simple sandwich of high-quality, low-glycemic bread like Ezekiel or Royo with almond butter will also work, as it will increase the fiber content in your gut, and the fat and protein provided by the almond butter will help delay the gastric emptying process.

FIGURE 4.4 Reactive Hypoglycemic Crash

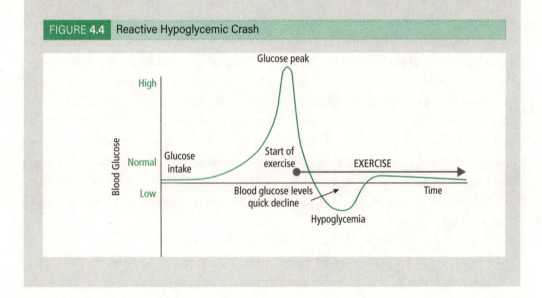

GLUCOSE STABILIZATION AND MAINTENANCE DURING YOUR WORKOUT OR EVENT

Your CGM will be of great use to you as you work out or compete. You'll be able to see exactly when your glucose begins to drop, how quickly (or slowly) it's dropping, and you'll be able to feed yourself correctly so that you can maintain your glucose levels within your GPZs. When you look at your CGM data every few minutes or you have live visibility of your glucose levels available alongside other performance parameters (heart rate, speed, power, pace, etc.), it will be very easy to manage your glucose levels within a relatively stable range, arrest any falling glucose levels times, increase your glucose levels when needed, and ensure that you've a steady supply of energy so that you can focus on your sport, whether that's a sport primarily using skills like basketball or soccer or an endurance sport like triathlon or cycling. This is one of the major advantages of CGM sensors: valuable real-time information about glucose concentration levels, direction, rate of change, and trends. All these parameters, not just the number itself, are important for decision-making.

Feeding and maintenance of glucose levels has been proven to enhance performance many times over, from increasing the accuracy of shots on goal in a soccer match to maintaining a steady wattage output in the Tour De France mountain stages.[44] There are many scientific studies that cover what kind of carbohydrates you should ingest, the grams per hour, and the science behind each claim, and that information is important to use and understand. Science teaches us the importance of fueling properly for athletic performance and it's very well known that even ingesting carbohydrates during a super intense one-hour workout can enhance performance. Feeding your muscles with glucose, which is converted into adenosine triphosphate (ATP), the energy of the cells, is critical for any super intense effort up to an hour. It becomes even more important after two and a half hours, as you'll have exhausted your liver and muscle glycogen stores.[45] Continued ingestion of carbohydrates is critical to continuing exercise at a level above endurance pace. What hasn't been studied is how important it is to: maintain stable blood glucose levels throughout the event, prevent the "roller coaster" of glucose levels, arrest the "slow slide" of a glucose drop, and not ingest too much too quickly (i.e., proper pacing of your foods and drinks). If you do your best to stabilize your glucose levels, this will stabilize your energy so you feel strong throughout your workout or event.

Your goal during exercise is to do your best to keep your glucose levels within your GPZ. That's not easy and sometimes you'll be on the roller coaster as you deal with the demands of your event or workout. However, with some careful planning and learning about your body's response to foods, you should be able to improve your ability to keep your glucose levels steady. Let's look at some glucose curves from different athletes so that you'll be able to recognize the same pattern if it happens to you and, therefore, make a change if need be or give yourself a pat on the back for a job well done!

Stable and Strong

In Figure 4.5, we see Peter Gasperini, an elite masters cyclist, age 58, who demonstrated a very good stable glucose level during a one-hour hill-climb time trial. Popularly known as a

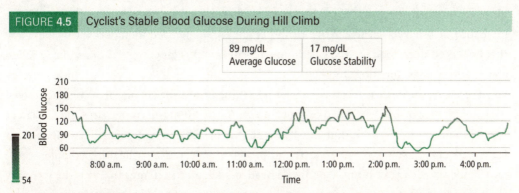

Peter Gasperini, an elite masters cyclist, age 58, who demonstrated a very good stable glucose level during a one-hour hill-climb time trial.

Functional Threshold Test (FTP), this effort was a full one-hour, all-out, do-your-best, at-the-highest-heart-rate-you-can-maintain, puke-at-the-end-of-it, kind of effort. Peter began riding at 10:30 a.m. that morning and rode for an hour to warm up. Notice how his glucose was very stable leading up to his ride (90 milligrams per deciliter (mg/dL) on average) and then increased (to 120 mg/dL) as he started riding. This was due to ingesting a glass of beet juice, which contains sugars, and helped to produce more power on the climb. As he rode, his glucose dropped (to 60 mg/dL). It's very typical to see a nice drop in glucose as you begin exercising and nothing to be concerned with. It happens as the pancreas releases more insulin than needed after an influx of sugars, and at the same time exercise begins. The body does not know that exercise is about to occur and then as the athlete begins exercising those sugars are taken up by the muscles, thereby causing a larger than needed drop in glucose. What's important for you to know here is that your blood glucose will come back up naturally as your liver releases more glucose into the bloodstream. Don't panic, it will come back up and stabilize, just as Peter's stabilized at about 11:45 a.m. He then had two sports gels, knowing that he needed to raise his glucose even higher, and right before he started his effort at 12:10 p.m., his glucose level came up to 145 mg/dL. As he began to push harder and harder, there was another initial drop to 90 mg/dL (again, no panicking here, this is normal and will come back up), followed by a rise to a range of 120–150 mg/dL. His liver was in overtime releasing glucose to be converted into energy for the muscles and the rest of the body. He continued to push at his FTP, finishing his one-hour time trial at 1:10 p.m., where his glucose level was right in his GPZ. The glucose stayed elevated afterward, as he had summited the climb and was resting at the top. You'll notice his glucose began to drop as he hadn't been replacing any of it along the way. His liver had stopped releasing any more, since his heart rate had come down and his pancreas was still releasing insulin and beginning to drive the glucose levels down. While he didn't feel like he needed food necessarily, he knew that he would need food for the ride home and to keep his glucose level up, so he grabbed some more sports nutrition and began pedaling home, which didn't require much energy and, therefore, the glucose levels went back up again, peaking at 154 mg/dL. When he arrived back home, his glucose levels had dropped down to the 60 mg/dL range since he didn't eat much lunch and it had been quite a while since his breakfast at 7:00 a.m. Thank goodness for a recovery shake of complex carbs and proteins, followed by a healthy, complex-carb-based lunch, which gave him the bump he needed back up to 120 mg/dL. With the recovery shake and food after his workout, insulin increased again and helped to shuttle those important nutrients into the cells for repair and recovery. So you *want* a spike after your hard workout. This is a great example of controlling blood glucose correctly for optimal performance *and* recovery.

The Roller Coaster

What happens when you do your best to stay stable, but you end up on the roller coaster? How does the roller coaster occur? There are, in general, three different scenarios in which you could create the roller coaster and for all of these, the roller coaster occurs in longer workouts (workouts that are over three hours) so this scenario typically only applies to endurance athletes.

The first scenario is the simplest. It's where you deliberately overeat simple carbs every 30 to 45 minutes or so, creating a massive glucose spike, not recognizing that you're dropping rapidly and then eating another large amount of simple carbs, and continuing this process. This is seen in athletes that are new to their sport and who have not figured out how to pace themselves during their training or competition from an intensity and fueling perspective. Of course, individual insulin sensitivity and training status also play a role. Most athletes will self-correct after they've done this a few times, as it's obvious that their energy levels are fluctuating wildly throughout their effort.

The second scenario is the more likely scenario, especially after you've been using your CGM for a little while and learn how to stabilize your glucose levels. This occurs when you're doing a longer workout, around four to five hours, and in the last one to two hours you run out of energy and just need something/anything to eat, as you've either not eaten correctly or you've eaten all the available food. In that last one to two hours, you drink a sugary soda or energy drink, eat some simple carbs, like fig bars, or sports gels or gummies, to get your glucose levels up quickly. In cases like this, where you're mildly low in glucose levels (hypoglycemic), you're nearing the end of a long workout, and you need that energy and glucose spike (and you need it now), it's likely you'll pick up a high-glycemic food to get you up again. This will however put you on the roller coaster. Once you're on the roller coaster, accept it and stay on it. The most important aspect of the roller coaster is that you've access to enough food so that you can continue to spike your glucose levels.

The third scenario is like the second scenario, but it comes in the last couple of days of a hard training block. Let's say you've been pushing the limits day in and day out for nearly two weeks. Your baseline glucose has dropped from 95 to 75 mg/dL. You've been eating like crazy yet still can't get enough carbs to truly replenish your glycogen stores and, in actuality, your glycogen stores are quite depleted from the start of your workout. You've no reserves, so you must rely entirely on the carbs you ingest for energy. See Figure 4.6. This is a common occurrence for cyclists that compete in cycling stage races where you have to compete day after day for up to 21 days, in something like the Tour de France, but it also occurs at the end of a hard training block. In this case, you're on the roller coaster right from the start of the workout. In Figure 4.7, we see my roller coaster that occurred at the end of a two-week block of hard training on the bicycle—up to five hours each day. This was the fourteenth day of training, and I was absolutely "on fumes" and in an over-reached state.

Figure 4.7 shows the last day of 2 weeks of hard training. I was riding on the edge of energy! Note, how much of a roller coaster this was. This is because my liver and muscle glycogen stores were low and I was basically operating on my blood glucose. The last three major spikes and drops were eating massive carbs in order to keep going, using those carbs as fuel and then needing more. Each of those drops had to be recognized and stopped with more food!

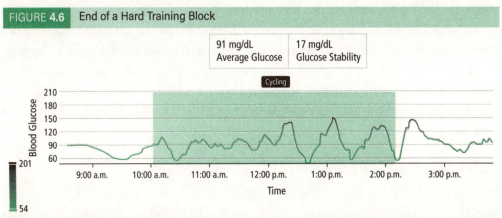

FIGURE 4.6 End of a Hard Training Block

Notice how the glucose values are generally below 120 mg/dL, with the peaks barely touching 150 mg/dL? These are much lower glucose levels than normal for me during a hard training ride. At the end of a hard training block, it is difficult to keep glucose levels high.

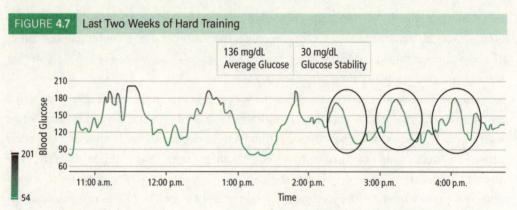

When you are low on glycogen stores at the end of a hard two-week cycle of training, it is difficult to maintain a stable level of glucose and you may often end up on a "roller coaster."

Right after my breakfast, my blood sugar went up to 200 mg/dL as I had a very carb-heavy breakfast, but it came down quickly as I was riding relatively intensely (tempo pace or over 80% of my FTP) and burning glucose—the little that I had on board. Within an hour of riding, I knew I had to eat very regularly on this training ride. I ate a sports bar, a banana, and pretzels, which stopped my drop at 90 mg/dL and brought it back up to 185 mg/dL. Within 30 minutes of that peak, I was crashing again having used all of that glucose. This time I couldn't stop the crash quite as quickly and my glucose levels dropped to 80 mg/dL, at which point I had to stop and get more food from the follow vehicle. This time, I ate three handfuls of trail mix, a small bag of chips, a protein bar, and two oranges. This gave me enough to keep going, as you can see from the third spike in the graph. The fourth, fifth and sixth spikes were similar, and I was able to just hang on for 30 to 45 minutes after each time I ate. At this point I knew I just had to keep shoveling as much food down as possible and it didn't matter too much what I had. I drank a soft drink and had a candy bar at the very end to give me the final boost to get done with the training, and that's the last spike on the right side of the graph. This obviously is *not* ideal, nor desired, and it's not much fun either! However, it can and will occur if you're training hard and long enough, so it's best that you recognize when you're on the roller coaster and just accept your fate. Keep eating and putting food in as much as possible.

Can you "get off" the roller coaster?

It's possible to get off the roller coaster and there are two guaranteed ways to do it. Number one: you can stop for an extended time (over 60 minutes) and eat a full meal that contains complex carbs, proteins, and fats. I recommend a ratio of 50/30/20 respectively, so that you slow down your digestive system and gastric emptying, which will help to stabilize your glucose levels.

Number two: you can continue exercising but eat more protein than carbs and only eat complex carbs, which are slower to digest. For example, you could eat three hard boiled eggs and a sweet potato or two, which would slow down your digestive system and give your body the carbs it needs to turn into glucose, but in a way that stabilizes and reduces your peaks and valleys in your glucose levels curve. Of course, you have to have access to those foods and/or a restaurant! The goal is to slow down your digestion and catch up on your caloric needs during your exercise.

The Cliff

The "cliff" occurs sometimes in your normal life right after a meal, where you experience a sharp increase in glucose levels followed by a sharp drop. This is usually normal and a good indication that you're insulin sensitive, and your body is dealing well with rises in glucose levels by reducing them quickly and getting you back to homeostasis or your baseline glucose. There is nothing to worry about here; it's a normal response. Not all spikes are bad (it depends on the context), and it's a myth that glucose needs to be stable 24/7.

In Figure 4.8 you can see this quick rise and fall, which is completely normal and nothing to worry about.

The cliff that is more concerning and what we want to avoid is the one that comes during training or competition. This only occurs after prolonged training, over two to two and a half hours, when you've used much of your stored glucose (glycogen) in the muscles and liver. Up to that point, your liver can release that

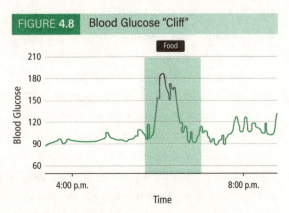

The "cliff" is a completely normal glucose response.

stored glycogen as glucose in your bloodstream so that you use it. Once this is depleted, it's likely you could have a sharp drop in glucose levels. This is a hypoglycemic crash or a "bonk" as cyclists call it. You can prevent this from happening by anticipating it and then eating before it occurs. Most endurance athletes begin eating an hour into exercise if they know they'll be exercising for over three hours, to prevent this crash from occurring. They will (and should) continue to eat every 30 to 45 minutes to ensure that ingested carbs are continuing to fuel muscles, sparing precious stored glycogen. Experimenting with a sports drink might help too: some anecdotal evidence from professional athletes shows that a continuous intake of carbs in liquid form rather that gels every 20 to 30 minutes causes a more stable glucose response. As you ingest glucose while exercising, your muscles quickly uptake and prefer these carbs to stored carbs for fuel. For endurance athletes that have long events (over four hours), the preservation of stored glycogen is critical so it can be used in the latter half of the event. Feeding yourself from near the beginning of your workout or event is a great way to preserve that glycogen for later. Of course, eating while exercising isn't always possible, and runners have the hardest time as it's challenging to eat and run at the same time! A glucose gel is an ideal product for runners, as it's easy to ingest and digest. It's important that you keep food around during your workouts or events, so that when you see this rapid drop (the cliff) in your glucose data and on your CGM, you can immediately ingest enough carbohydrates. I would also suggest that you make a mental note of it, to prevent it happening again. In Figure 4.9, we see a triathlete doing a long run where she had her glucose levels at a high level for a long time (nearly three hours) and then a big crash at the end of the workout.

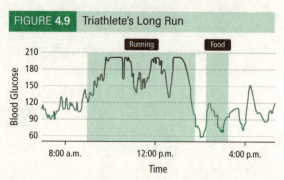

Sustaining a high level of glucose during exercise is challenging because you could "crash" without much warning.

The other way it happens is when you have high glucose levels for an extended time and then you stop exercising. Your pancreas takes some time to catch up after you've stopped exercising, as your muscle cells are still sending signals to uptake as much glucose as possible. Your pancreas will continue to release enough insulin to reduce all the remaining high glucose levels in your bloodstream. These two things combined can cause a sudden drop in blood glucose. This can be a disconcerting feeling, and you could feel dizzy, shaky, and quite possibly panicky—these are symptoms of a hypoglycemic crash. You might be confused as to why this is happening since you had a higher level of glucose very recently and now you feel like you're bonking! Watch out for this phenomenon. The solution here is to ingest food, specifically complex carbs with protein, to help stabilize the glucose levels without spiking it again.

Example of a normal drop of glucose during workouts

What is "normal?" A question many a philosopher has asked over the millennia! In terms of glucose levels, it's also hard to define what is normal, but there are many reoccurring patterns that show up during exercise. For example, after eating a healthy breakfast of complex-carb cereal, like muesli, with almond milk, berries, and one tablespoon of almond butter, martial artist and motorcycle coach, Aaron Stevenson's glucose levels increased his fasting glucose levels of 70 mg/dL in the morning to 120 mg/dL, and stabilized there just before his martial art workout. Within 15 minutes of the start of his workout, his glucose levels began dropping and continued down until reaching 60 mg/dL. They then began to climb back up, reaching 75 mg/dL at the end of his workout. After his workout, his glucose levels rose again, to 120 mg/dL, and remained stable for the next one and a half hours.

This is a normal response to a workout. Aaron's glucose levels had risen because of his breakfast, then once he began exercising, the circulating glucose levels began rapidly being shuttled into the muscle cells to be used for energy creation, thereby quickly reducing the circulating glucose levels. This looks like a hypoglycemic crash, but it's not. This is where you need to understand the circumstances and context around your glucose levels and learn what is a hypo crash and what is a normal response. Both look the same, but they're not. In Figure 4.10 the glucose levels began to rise after about 30 minutes of intense martial arts, as Aaron had presumably used much of his ingested carbs and it could have been possible (although we don't know for sure) that his liver had begun releasing more to take up the slack in the bloodstream.

After his workout, his glucose levels continued back up to the 120 mg/dL mark because the need for glucose levels had stopped and his food was still digesting, releasing more glucose

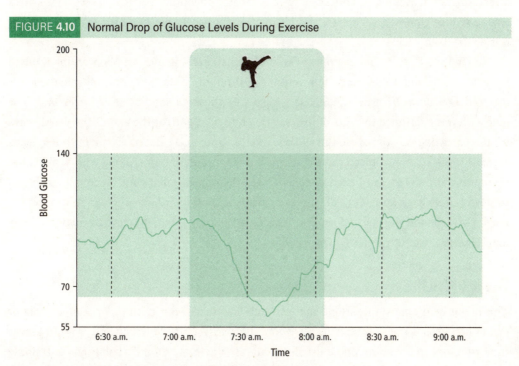

FIGURE 4.10 Normal Drop of Glucose Levels During Exercise

A normal and expected drop in glucose levels from exercise after a meal.

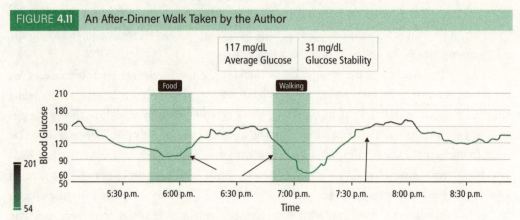

A walk after your meal can make a big difference in lowering your glucose levels.

into his bloodstream. His glucose levels stabilized at 120 mg/dL afterward, as his body continued to digest the food and circulate the glucose levels.

Let's look at a relatively nonathletic exercise (walking) where this "normal" drop occurs, so you can better understand that this is a normal response to exercise. Many people take walks after dinner each evening and this is something I would encourage you to do as well. It's a great way to reduce glucose level spikes, and it's just a great way to get in a little extra movement during the day.

In Figure 4.11, this is an example of when I had an evening meal of Mexican food, raised my glucose levels up to 150, and then went for a 30-minute walk. Note how my glucose levels dropped as soon as I began walking, as I was using those glucose levels as I exercised. The glucose levels continued to drop all the way down to 63 mg/dL at the end of the walk! Wow, what an amazing way to reduce the glucose levels in your body and use some of those sugars you just ingested. Now, since I did eat a *large* burrito, beans, and rice, along with some chips, there was more sugar than I needed, so as soon as I stopped walking my glucose levels began to slowly climb back up 150 mg/dL and even peaked at 160 mg/dL, nearly two hours after my meal. This rebound rise is also normal and nothing to worry about, it's more a function of how many grams of carbohydrates you ingested!

THE SLOW SLIDE

This might be the most important one to watch for during your training or competition, or just in life. I call it the slow slide because your glucose levels slide slowly down over a longer time, from one to five hours, and it usually occurs after at least two and a half hours of training or competing. It might start out at 140 mg/dL while you're in your GPZ, and then after some

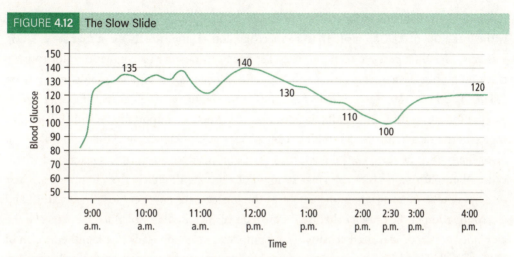

Recognizing the slow slide during exercise is critical to preventing hypoglycemia and maintaining a peak performance.

extended time exercising you see it drop down to 135, then to 130, 125, 120, 115, 110, 105, 100, etc., and this could take place over a period of three hours. You feel fine, you feel fine, you're training or competing well, and then out of the blue you feel hungry, and you need to eat right away! Well, of course, this wasn't out of the blue, it happened over the past three hours and in a slow slide. This slide was quite possibly so slow that you didn't really notice it because you were so intensely focused on your sport. This is exactly why it's quite possibly one of the most important patterns for you to recognize as you train or compete. Once you begin to pay attention to your glucose levels, and you start to see this pattern happen, then you'll know that you can easily address it by ingesting just enough carbs to slowly begin pushing it back up. The critical thing here is that you don't overeat carbs and create a reactive hypoglycemic crash (read further for more on this). I recommend that you start with 15–20 g of carbs and then wait some time, around five minutes or 10 minutes, and see what your glucose levels do. If they don't come up, then have another 15–20 g of carbs and that should do it. Again, give it five or 10 minutes and see what your CGM reports. In Figure 4.12, the cyclist was doing a long race that was over six hours long, and the slow slide began around 11:30 a.m. after two and a half hours of racing. That slide continued until 2:30 p.m. as the glucose levels reached 100 mg/dL down from 140 mg/dL at 11:30 a.m. At this point, the athlete ingested carefully and began to raise and stabilize their glucose levels.

THE REACTIVE HYPO CRASH

This is something we all want to avoid, and it's a critical one to understand. This is something that we, the athlete, actually create! Some individuals are more susceptible to developing a rebound hypo than others for reasons unknown at this point. We do this to ourselves, and without the use of a CGM, it's hard to connect the dots that we are the ones that are creating this crash. Here's a possible scenario: A cyclist has been racing in a competition for roughly three hours but hasn't been eating enough and is in the midst of a slow slide, going from 135 mg/dL down to 80 mg/dL. Finally realizing that their glucose levels are getting dangerously low (for them), reaching 80 mg/dL, they panic as they know an important deciding hill is coming up in the race in about 45 minutes. They jam six gummy blocks into their mouth, which gives them 48 g of carbs (200 kilocalories (k/cals)), mostly from simple sugars, and which causes their glucose levels to rise from 80 mg/dL to 160 mg/dL in less than 10 minutes. Their muscles uptake these sugars immediately, as the muscles are now very insulin sensitive, and the contraction of the muscles themselves are a powerful stimulator of glucose uptake. So the combined action of increased sensitivity and muscle contraction leads to a rapid reduction of glucose in the blood. This causes a reactive hypoglycemic crash, where the glucose levels drop even *lower* than before, down to 60 mg/dL. This cyclist now feels like they're bonking again, and even worse than the first time!

See Figure 4.13. Without having a CGM, the cyclist incorrectly assumes they didn't take in enough carbs, so they eat another six gummy blocks, trying to get the glucose levels back up again, and now the roller coaster has started! Had this cyclist been using a CGM, firstly, they would have recognized the slow slide and stopped the glucose levels from getting too low and,

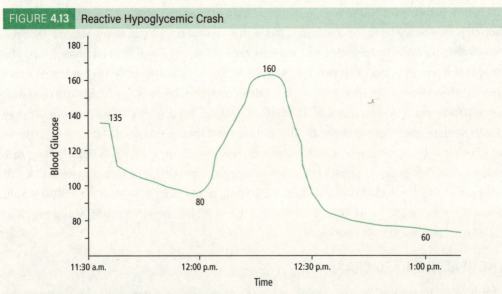

FIGURE 4.13   Reactive Hypoglycemic Crash

Many athletes do not realize that they are creating a "bonk," or reactive hypoglycemic crash, by ingesting too many carbohydrates too quickly during exercise.

CHAPTER 4: Using a CGM for Optimal Training, Competing, and Recovery   67

secondly, they would have known that the better strategy was to eat two to three of the gummy blocks, sucking on them for three to four minutes before chewing them and swallowing, allowing for a three to five minute time lag, and observing if that was enough to get their glucose levels back up without creating a large spike. If the glucose levels don't start coming back up after that six-to-nine-minute period, they would take out two more gummy blocks, suck on them and then chew them and wait another three to five minutes before repeating again. This way, the athlete can better control the rise in glucose levels, so that it gradually comes back up and does *not* create a large spike followed by a large crash—the reactive hypo crash. The timing of this is highly individual due to the different insulin sensitivities that people have, so keep that in mind as it could be 10 minutes for you and 15 minutes for a friend. When you use your CGM, create the reactive hypo crash for yourself, see how it works, and the epiphany will occur! It's truly mind-blowing for many endurance athletes to realize that the reactive hypo crash is something that *they* are creating themselves! For years and years (in fact, one of the first papers to measure glucose at the end of exercise was in 1924) athletes have been warned about "the crash," but not until the advent of CGMs have they been able to realize just how many of these crashes are reactive hypo crashes that they have created unknowingly.[46]

IDEAL GLUCOSE LEVELS DURING A WORKOUT OR EVENT

Now that I've given you some examples of what can happen if things don't go exactly as planned, have a read of what could be considered as an ideal glucose level profile for a workout or event. As written previously, keeping a stable glucose level value throughout your workout is something to strive for. You might never achieve it though. In over two and a half years of using a CGM in competitions, workouts, cycling camps, long hikes—you name it—I have had little success in maintaining perfectly stable glucose levels; yet, I've performed well on most occasions. This doesn't mean that the ideal isn't achievable, just because I haven't been able to get it perfect. You can still perform well with a little more fluctuation within the exercise. The key is in understanding the previous scenarios and making sure you know what to do, or *not* do, when you see them. On the other hand, I've seen hundreds and hundreds of nearly ideal glucose level curves from athletes in their chosen sport, so it's possible to keep your glucose stable during training and competition. Not only do these athletes maintain solid and stable glucose levels values but they also perform at high levels with great success.

By keeping your glucose levels stable, you'll have a more consistent workout, your energy levels won't fade, you'll be more mentally alert, and you'll just feel better throughout the event. Again, the goal is to maintain as stable glucose levels as possible, for you. Your glucose levels might fluctuate a lot more than a training partner's, and that's perfectly fine. There's also a difference between male and female responses. A recent paper showed a small difference in

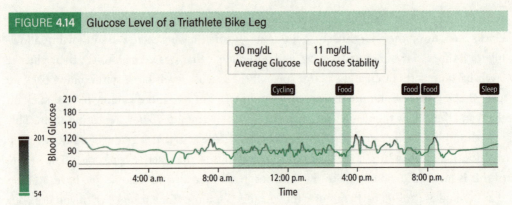

This triathlete kept her glucose values stable throughout the triathlon by ingesting the right kind of carbs at the right time.

glucose response in females compared to males—females are generally lower than males (check Figure 4 in their paper).[47] The opposite could also be the case. Maybe your levels are always stable and it seems no matter how many grams of carbohydrates you ingest, nothing moves your glucose number. That is also perfectly fine, and I would argue that this is a characteristic of a slow responder, as we talked about earlier in this chapter.

Let's look at three different graphs showing stable glucose level curves during exercise. In Figure 4.14, you'll see a stable curve from a triathlete during a 70.3 triathlon race. This triathlete kept her glucose levels very stable for the entire bike leg, averaging 90 mg/dL. There were some slight fluctuations in the glucose, but they were so minor. This was impressive stability. She drank one bottle of UCAN® with 60 g of carbs and had two sports gels, one about half way and then another with just a quarter of the bike leg to go. She had one of her very best bike leg splits and went on to run a PR in her run leg.

In the next example you'll see a bodybuilder, Lorenzo Elder, who does a strength workout for nearly two hours. Notice that during his weightlifting workout, his glucose levels were extremely stable. This appears to be very low in comparison to many athletes, but this is his normal level, and he can perform fine all day long at 70 mg/dL, which for most people would be categorized as mild hypoglycemia. He sipped on a sports drink throughout his two-hour heavy session and maintained incredibly stable glucose levels. This is just one of many examples of weightlifters/bodybuilders that I have where their glucose levels are very stable during workouts. At the time of publishing, there are no studies on weightlifters and blood glucose levels, or with CGM data, so I can only postulate that two things are occurring here. Firstly, weightlifters have so much muscle mass that glucose is soaked up immediately in the muscle, keeping the circulating glucose lower; and secondly, their heart rates stay low during weight training, and therefore the sympathetic nervous system reduces glucose production.[48]

In Figure 4.15, we can see a bodybuilder's incredible glucose stability throughout the day, including the weight session.

Our last example of stability during a workout or event is by an avid pickleball player. Scott Cohen gets up early every other day during the week, and goes to play pickleball with his buddies at the local court. He's an intense player and has heart rates into the 150 beats per minute during matches. He plays at this intensity level for about an hour each time. In this scenario, Scott has not eaten anything since the previous night's dinner at around 7:00 p.m. Therefore, he is using the stored muscle and liver glycogen to exercise at this intensity.

In Figure 4.16, his glucose levels increased just a little from 90 mg/dL to 100 mg/dL during the match and then began to drop toward the end of the hour, to 85 mg/dL. His body kept his glucose levels in tight control for his workout, and since it was only one hour long, he had

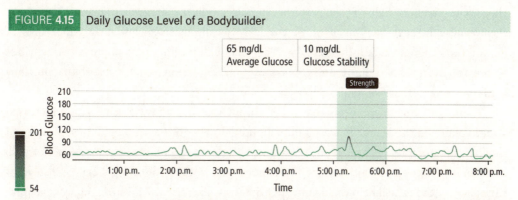

Bodybuilder Lorenzo Elder's daily glucose level is low when compared to most people, including during his weightlifting sessions. However, his body performs well at these below-average levels.

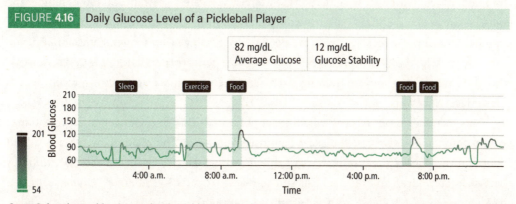

Scott Cohen keeps his glucose levels stable throughout most of the day, and an early-morning intense pickleball game does not impact his glucose levels.

plenty of stored muscle and liver glycogen to use. After showering, which produced a fake spike, or "artifact" (reminder: abrupt changes in temperature can give you false data), he went to his favorite restaurant for a healthy breakfast, which raised his glucose levels to 120 mg/dL, but only briefly. Then it appeared he had a reactive hypo crash, but we know this is not the case. It was just his body doing its best to regulate insulin and glucose levels, and we can see his glucose levels stabilized later at 10:00 a.m. He then had a "slow slide" all the way to dinner, as he often skips lunch.

POST-TRAINING OR EVENT RECOVERY

After your workout or competition, you can use your CGM to better understand if you're getting the correct blood glucose response, to help you improve your recovery. The goal of any post-exercise recovery shake, meal, or snack is to replenish the nutrients that you used during your event. They also help to rapidly restore muscle and liver glycogen stores so that you have less soreness the next day, you adapt more quickly to training stress, and most importantly of all, you can train hard again the next day. The goal of all training is to improve performance through an overload of training stress, followed by an adaptation to that stress so that previous load is no longer stressful.

There are many adaptations that occur throughout the body, which include increased stroke volume in the heart, increased mitochondrial mass, increased muscle mass, improved capillarization of muscles, and so on. These adaptations are specific to the exercises performed. Want to be a better bodybuilder? Spending more time in the gym lifting weights, instead of running marathons, will help you adapt. High-intensity exercise will give you different adaptations than low-intensity exercise. Resistance training with heavy weights and a low number of reps will give you a different adaptation than going to a CrossFit gym, where you might do hundreds of reps with light weights.[49] Every exercise will cause a certain amount of fatigue and muscle soreness and stiffness after a workout or multiple days of workouts. Your goal is to minimize this downtime, so that you can get back to training again sooner. For example, if you can only train hard on two days a week, but your competitors train hard for four days a week, they'll be able to create more training stress, and therefore more adaptations, resulting in a higher level than you.

This section will not tell you which exact potion to drink or secret snack bar to eat after your workouts, nor give you the exact quantities you need. There are many other excellent books on the market that are better to help you with that. I recommend *Sport Nutrition* by Dr. Asker Jeukendrup and Michael Gleeson, along with *Sports Nutrition for Endurance Athletes* by Monique Ryan, which are both excellent and comprehensive.

Post-Workout Glucose Spike

There have been hundreds of studies on the optimal post-workout food, shake, or meal. Almost all of them have found that at least 60 g of carbohydrates will give you a glucose spike and then cause insulin to be released. What you're trying to do is to get enough insulin into the system, so that it can "open the door" to the cells for glucose and proteins, vitamins and other nutrients to go in and repair muscle damage and replenish glycogen stores. The cells are very insulin sensitive after exercise, so they rapidly uptake glucose from the blood and store it as glycogen. It is a bit of a catch-22 scenario, in that you need glucose to go into the cells, but in order for this to happen you need insulin. Without glucose there is no insulin, and without insulin the glucose can't enter the cells. The great news is that post-workout and competition shakes and meals usually taste great!

There is plenty of evidence proving that just a carbohydrate solution post-exercise will cause a sufficient release of insulin. However, I recommend a carbohydrate to protein blend, as post-workout you're also repairing muscle and helping muscle synthesis, or the formation of new muscle cells. A recovery drink that contains a ratio of anywhere between 4:1 to 2:1 (carb/protein) should be sufficient to stimulate an insulin release and also provide amino acids. Personally, I like a 2:1 (carb/protein) ratio, as I want to ensure that I'm giving my muscles enough amino acids, including the very important leucine, after a workout.[50] The amount that you need depends on the length and intensity of your workout. The longer and more intense the workout, the greater the need for more calories overall. A five-hour bike ride over two mountain passes where you burn over 3000 k/cals, will require you to drink a large recovery shake and eat a full and well-balanced meal in the two hours after. The shorter and less intense the workout, the lower the need. If you do a one-hour intense workout, you may or may not even need a post-workout recovery shake or meal.

Using 1.0–1.5 g of carbs per kg of body weight and 0.8–1.2 g of protein per kg of body weight will be sufficient. Going with the high end of carbs and the low end of protein, this would work out at 105 g of carbs and 56 g of protein in the two hours after a workout. Monique Ryan, MS, RDN, CSSD and the author of *Sports Nutrition for Endurance Athletes* said, "A diet adequate in carbohydrate is superior for recovery from training and replenishing muscle glycogen stores. Nutritional recovery takes place from one training session to the next. After moderate to hard training sessions, nutritional recovery can be jump-started with 1.2 g carbohydrate per kilogram of body weight within the 30–60 minutes after training. This rapid phase of carbohydrate recovery is especially important if the next training session takes place in less than 12 hours. The total carbohydrate requirements for the day can range from 5 to 7 g/kg weight for moderate short training sessions and low-intensity endurance training; increasing

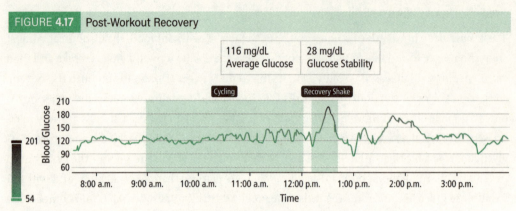

An ideal post-workout recovery glucose spike from a recovery shake and meal.

to 6–10 g/kg for moderate to heavy endurance training of up to three hours; with the highest needs at 8–12 g/kg for hard endurance training lasting over three hours."[51]

In Figure 4.17, the athlete did a Functional Threshold Test (FTP), which is a one-hour all-out on a bicycle, in the middle of the workout. This athlete stopped before his FTP test, took two gels of 22 g of carbs each and then rode easy to the start of the test. You can see that his glucose levels were on the upswing when he started the test, indicating perfect priming for this super-intense effort, and it continued to stay high throughout the test.

After the test, his glucose levels returned to within his normal, endurance pace GPZ as he cruises home. Once at home, he drank a recovery shake with carbs and protein in the right ratio suggested above, and this resulted in a perfect post-workout recovery glucose spike right after the workout stopped. He cooled off, stretched, took a shower, and made a healthy meal. Roughly 60 minutes after completing his workout, he has another spike that comes from a post-workout recovery meal. This is the optimal glucose profile you're aiming for to give yourself the best chance at recovering for the following day. It also helps you take all that training stress and adapt to become stronger.

Let's look a little closer at Figure 4.17. Notice that the recovery shake spike goes up to 190 mg/dL and then comes down to about 85 mg/dL in less than 30 minutes. His cells are more insulin sensitive and soak up all the glucose he has ingested. At the same time, he has a big insulin release (which is what you want) so that he can get in as much glucose, proteins, and nutrients into his cells. This pulls the glucose out of the bloodstream, leading to a mild reactive hypoglycemic crash afterward. It's not really a low blood-sugar crash, but merely a reaction, and should give you confirmation that your recovery shake is doing its job.

Now, have a look at the second spike after his meal around 1:30 p.m. This has a completely different shape, where it does not peak as high, and it lasts longer than the very "peaky" recovery shake. It's most likely that he had ingested enough carbs, and his glycogen stores had reached the maximum of what they could store at this point. (They'll be able to store more, but through later meals.) This should give you confidence that, indeed, you've taken in enough carbs after your workout to replenish your glycogen stores and optimize the recovery and repair process. The second spike also most likely indicates slower gastric emptying, as presumably his meal contained fiber from vegetables, healthy proteins, and healthy fats from olive oil. Either way, the two shapes of these curves are what you want. This is what you're striving to create in your post-workout/competition nutrition protocol.

IN SUMMARY

After reading this chapter, you should have a better understanding of the different shapes of glucose responses: what causes them, how to create the response you want for the right situation, and what are both ideal and not so ideal scenarios. Clearly, it's complicated stuff. With so many variables influencing the glucose response, it truly is something personal to you. What's important is that you learn these responses to enhance your athletic performance. This will involve understanding why they are occurring, what to do (if anything), and how to manipulate them to optimize your pre-workout/competition priming and your fueling during your workout/competition. With this insight you'll be able to create the best strategy for post-workout recovery and repair.

CHAPTER 5

Strategies on CGM Use for Performance

BLOOD GLUCOSE LEVELS ARE COMPLICATED—we know that by now—but one thing that really sticks out when looking at all of these glucose curves is the constant fluctuations. You never see a perfectly flat line, and very rarely do you see a line that just fluctuates 2–3 milligrams per deciliter (mg/dL). Your body is an ever-changing organism that is constantly trying to maintain some level of homeostasis within millions of different systems and cells. It's a miracle that blood glucose is as stable as it is, to be honest! To better understand and quantify this seemingly random fluctuating line, we'll dig into the key terms you should know and look at what the curves mean, so that you can better interpret your data. After you can interpret and understand the curves, then you can make decisions, if needed, on how to change the timing of your food intake, the types of food you eat, and even how much you eat.

AVERAGE GLUCOSE

This is simply the average glucose across a certain time range. This is very useful in a couple of respects. Firstly, when you create a "range" around a particular interest point, such as a meal, you learn your average blood glucose for that time frame. When you do this, it's important to begin your range from when you started eating, across the peak value, and back to when your blood glucose stabilizes. This way you capture the average for the entire time the food affected your blood glucose. This also applies when you exercise: be sure to create a "range" from the start of your training to the end. Secondly, I also believe it's important to learn the average blood glucose for your sleep, so I encourage you to create a range around your sleep every morning. If you're below 100 mg/dL, that's good; below 90 mg/dL is even better. If you're at 65 mg/dL, that's likely too low and you're in a calorie deficit. You might not be fueling enough to help with your recovery. Third, your average glucose for the entire day is also important to watch. When your average blood glucose for the day is 100 mg/dL or less,

AN IMPORTANT NOTE ON DAILY AVERAGE GLUCOSE

Since you're an athlete and working out most likely six hours or more per week, you'll be burning more calories than most people. This means that you'll also need to be refueling more than most people. For the average person, an average daily glucose under 100 mg/dL is a good number, but since you're an athlete, you could easily exceed this, but not have to worry. Imagine if you work out intensely for three hours and your blood glucose stays within your glucose performance zone (GPZ) of 140–165 mg/dL for this entire time. Certainly, this will skew your daily average glucose high and could easily push you into the 115–120 mg/dL daily average range, where a normal person could be diagnosed as a prediabetic. You, however, know better, so keep this in mind when reviewing your daily averages.

that's good and means that you most likely don't have any prediabetic tendencies. If you're seeing over 120 mg/dL, I would suggest connecting with your primary care physician to learn if you're at risk of type 2 diabetes, or are already diabetic, and then take the appropriate steps.

GLUCOSE STABILITY OR VARIABILITY

This is the height (amplitude) and drop of your glucose, averaged over a certain time. The standard deviation or variability refers to the fluctuations in your glucose levels throughout the day, or across an event or exercise. Lower variability indicates a more stable and controlled blood glucose. It's measured by calculating how much your glucose varies from your average reading in mg/dL. A stable day with fewer fluctuations results in lower variability, while more significant fluctuations lead to higher variability.

Whenever you create a range around the event, this will give you the stability or variability of that event. This is useful over a longer time, around three or more hours, overnight, or for your entire day. The goal here is to reduce the number so that you've more stability and less variability. Some continuous glucose monitor (CGM) company apps call this "stability" and others call it "variability," so it's important to understand which one means what. However, the goal is to reduce your blood glucose number. For example, if I've a day where I'm traveling and haven't planned well, I'll need to eat out at restaurants and, therefore, it's very difficult to control my blood glucose. My average for the day might be 98 mg/dL and my variability might be 24 mg/dL. This means that the average over the entire day of "ups and downs" in my glucose curve was +/− 24 mg/dL from the average of 98 mg/dL. Not bad, but not great either, as this most likely means I had some big spikes that went up by 60 mg/dL in between my normal basal level of 95–100 mg/dL per day. Contrast this with a day in the office, where I can easily control my food options, eat as I need to and when I want to. My average for a day like this might be 83 mg/dL and my variability might be 12 mg/dL. So a day with much smaller rises and falls keeps my blood glucose more stable. Reducing my variability by 50% is a huge improvement for health and energy levels, not to mention mood.

The Levels company has a Stability Score, which "provides a quick overview of how stable your glucose levels were on a given day and allows you to track the trend of your stability day over day. It is represented on a scale of 60 to 100, you can think of this like a letter grade, where a higher score indicates more stable glucose levels. The score is influenced by the duration of stable glucose periods with fewer spikes. Levels' spike algorithm continuously monitors and detects significant glucose excursions in real time, prompting you to take action to mitigate spikes and observe how your glucose responds."[52]

Is there an optimal amount of variability you're aiming for? From an athletic perspective, if you do a short workout, say less than two hours, this metric has no real meaning. It's just not a long enough workout to cause your liver and muscle glycogen stores to be depleted, so there should be little intake of glucose during the workout, which in turn would cause a higher variability. For a longer workout, over three or four hours, when the muscle and liver glycogen stores are significantly decreased, and you need to ingest carbohydrates, then do your best to keep this under 20 mg/dL.

For individuals without obesity or diabetes, a normal average magnitude of glucose excursions (the difference between high and low points) falls between 26 and 28 mg/dL. To maintain lower variability, it's recommended not to exceed a 30 mg/dL rise from your pre-meal glucose levels, with a post-meal value not exceeding 110 mg/dL.

TIME OVER AND TIME UNDER

The amount of time spent over a specified glucose value, and put into "buckets" each hour of the day, is an excellent way to visualize when exactly your blood glucose is at its lowest throughout the day and when you have higher values. This can help you in a couple of ways as an athlete. In the mornings, nearly everyone will have the lowest value of the day, so if you tend to work out early in the morning, it's important to ensure that you've enough glucose on board to get in a strong workout. If you exercise right after you finish your work at 5:00 p.m., but you notice that's a really low time for your blood glucose, then ensuring that you increase your blood glucose with a healthy snack before your workout to "prime" yourself, will make a difference in the quality of your workout. Of course, make sure you prime with the right timing and have food nearby so that you can keep your blood glucose in your

GPZ for the workout. In Figure 5.0, we see a distribution chart of a triathlete's glucose over six months. This shows the number of times her glucose was less than 70mg/dL across the 24-hour day. Clearly, her glucose goes below 70mg/dL many times in the early morning hours, which is fine and expected. However, more concerning is the amount of times it dips below 70mg/dL from 4:00 p.m. to 8:00 p.m., which is when she trains. She would most likely benefit from raising her glucose levels before her workouts.

In Figure 5.1, we see at what times during the day this athlete goes over 140mg/dL across two years of data. Clearly, this athlete's lunch causes a glucose bump every day, followed by a slide of glucose levels leading into dinner. Dinner also has a significant impact on his glucose levels, so he should make sure he eats early to give his body a chance to reduce glucose levels by bedtime. Based on these glucose levels, his best time to workout would be after digesting his lunch when his glucose levels are the highest.

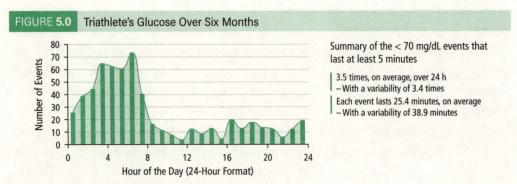

FIGURE 5.0 Triathlete's Glucose Over Six Months

The time during the day spent under 70 mg/dL, over a six-month period.

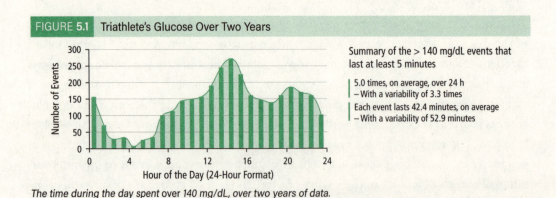

FIGURE 5.1 Triathlete's Glucose Over Two Years

The time during the day spent over 140 mg/dL, over two years of data.

WHAT DO ALL THESE SQUIGGLY LINES MEAN?

So, what is a good blood glucose response after a meal? What about during a workout? Can you tell if your liver and muscle cells are jam-packed with glycogen? What if your blood glucose is really low all the time? These are all great questions and as you continue your journey to learn more about your blood glucose curves, you'll most likely ask these questions, and more. I attempt to answer as many of these as possible so that you'll be able to recognize your response and interpret it correctly. In Chapter 8, you'll learn about how to use a CGM to increase your longevity and vitality, so it's likely some of your questions about your glucose curves will be answered there, like: How can I tell if I've prediabetes, or another issue? What should I be concerned about? What does that curve look like? What's a good response to a big ingestion of glucose?

There are so many thousands of different scenarios to consider that it's beyond the scope of this book to illustrate them all. I'll be putting many additional curves and case studies on my website: www.TrainingandCompetingwithCGM.com. Lastly, a gentle reminder: your blood glucose might not fit any of these curves. As I wrote in Chapter 4, there are so many factors which influence your blood glucose. You'll sometimes scratch your head when you see something that spikes your blood glucose that didn't spike it two days ago. Keep an open and inquisitive mind as you continue your pursuit of excellence.

What Is a Good Blood Glucose Response After a Meal?

The response you're looking for after a meal that contains carbohydrates is a spike that goes up and then quickly comes down. See Figure 5.2. The lower the spike, the better, of course, but this is largely dependent on the type and quality of the carbs in your meal. If you've a lot of simple, refined flours and sugars in your meal, your blood glucose spike will go much higher than if you've more complex carbs and fiber. As written earlier, a lower spike is better as it's less inflammatory to the body (anything over 140 mg/dL is considered inflammatory).[53] What is even more important, though, is how quickly your body brings you back to your base line or homeostasis. A quick return to baseline means that you've great insulin sensitivity.

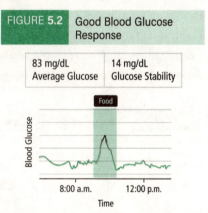

A quick rise, release of insulin, and then reduction back to baseline shows good insulin sensitivity.

What's a Response You Should Be Concerned About?

It could be a cause for concern if your blood glucose goes over 130 mg/dL and stays up for a long time—anywhere from one and a half hours to three hours. This means that you quite possibly have some insulin resistance. Now, the caveats to this are many, so don't panic. One of the scenarios in which your blood glucose will stay high for a longer period, but most likely doesn't indicate any issues, is when you've a large meal that also contains proteins and fats in equal amounts. These will slow the gastric emptying process and could possibly keep the blood glucose high for a long period of time. More concerning is if you quite frequently have meals where it takes hours for your blood glucose to reduce.

You should also be concerned if your baseline is over 110 mg/dL.[54] If your baseline is high and you have done a finger-stick test to ensure your CGM is reading correctly, then you should probably have that checked out. I recently was coaching an athlete whose baseline was 120 mg/dL. As soon as I saw their data, I knew they needed to see a doctor. Sure enough, their hemoglobin (HbA1C) was 6.7 and their fasting glucose was 115 mg/dL, and they were placed on a prescription drug to help bring it down. The good news is that with a change in diet, where they began a more whole-food plant-based diet, more awareness of their food intake, and additional weight loss and training, they were able to bring their HbA1c down to 5.4, and fasting glucose down to 95 mg/dL.

In Figure 5.3, this CrossFit athlete's glucose shows that they ate some food at 4:30 p.m., which raised their glucose to 120 mg/dL, where it stayed until nearly 7:00 p.m. This is quite a long time for their glucose to remain this high, especially since they were just in the office being sedentary. Their insulin resistance shows up again at dinner at 7:15 p.m. with a bump to nearly 180 mg/dL. Their glucose levels then stay over 120 mg/dL until 9:30 p.m., when it drops down and they start to feel hungry again. Eating a snack at 10:00 p.m. before bed shoots their

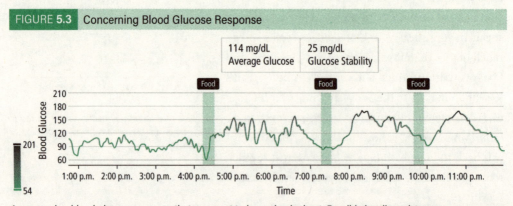

FIGURE 5.3 Concerning Blood Glucose Response

A concerning blood glucose response that you want to have checked out. Possible insulin resistance.

glucose back up to nearly 180 mg/dL, and it is still at 120 mg/dL when they go to bed. These are the slow returns back to "post meal baseline" that should be concerning. If you have a fast return, as seen in Figure 5.2, you should not be concerned. But if you are experiencing these slower returns, you may need to have this checked out.

What About When Your Blood Glucose Goes Up, but Not Too High, and Stays Stable for a Long Time?

This scenario is similar to the previous one, but your blood glucose goes from 90 mg/dL, for example, to 115 mg/dL and stays there for three to four hours before returning to 90 mg/dL. It makes a nice smooth sloping transition to 115 mg/dL and then a nice sloping descent back to 90 mg/dL. This is an example of eating a very good meal with plenty of fiber from vegetables, beans and greens, complex carbs, and healthy, low-fat proteins. I would argue that this is something you should strive for every day in your meals. Increasing your blood glucose to a little over your baseline, gives your cells the glucose they need, before then slowly coming back down. The example in Figure 5.4 also demonstrates why interpreting your glucose curves can be misleading and challenging. If you do not understand the context of the glucose responds, then you could think that this athlete has insulin resistance. In this case, this athlete has a very normal baseline glucose level, eats an above average healthy diet, and understands at a very advanced level how to manipulate their glucose level to give them the energy they need when they need it. Figure 5.4 shows a late dinner followed by an active evening of dancing and concert listening.

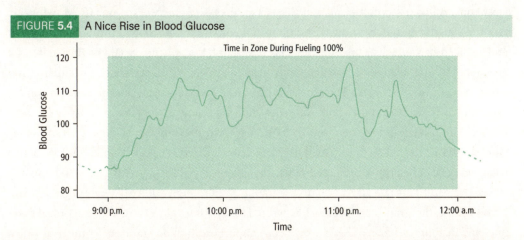

FIGURE 5.4 A Nice Rise in Blood Glucose

A nice rise, but not too much, extended stable glucose, and a slow return to baseline indicates that this athlete ate some complex carbs and a good blend of proteins and fats to sustain them for a longer time with higher baseline levels.

How Do You Know Your Glycogen Stores Are Completely Topped Off? Did You Carbo Load?

After a prolonged period of training or competing over multiple days, you'll find it harder and harder to restore your glycogen stores and, eventually, cumulative fatigue will set in and you'll find yourself in a nonfunctional, over-reaching state, where you can still train but you continue to become more and more fatigued. The only solution is rest and recover. How long should you recover? There have been many studies on this, along with complex mathematical algorithms and software to help understand when you're fully recovered. I worked for many years analyzing power data from cycling and using such a software tool, called the Performance Manager Chart, which quantifies training load. This tool was created by Dr. Andrew R. Coggan and integrated in the www.TrainingPeaks.com software and is a great tool to help you understand when to rest or train more. Like blood glucose responses, the answer to this question is multifactorial and complicated, depending on each situation, rider, and training load. One of the characteristics of an athlete that is fully recovered and ready for hard training again, is that their blood glucose will rise higher than normal. They'll have completely filled their muscle and liver glycogen stores to the top, and will begin to "overflow." What this means, practically, is that after a period of rest (the length of time can be different for each person), the athlete will start to see they've much higher blood glucose levels than their usual base levels, and their blood glucose spikes will also be higher than normal, along with a slower return to baseline. It will appear that they've acquired some insulin resistance all of the sudden! What is happening, though, is just like if you had a full tank of gas in your car, but you keep pumping and forcing more gas into the tank, this will cause the gas to spill over. The same thing is happening in your body. All your stores are full and there is an excess of glucose, so your CGM will begin reporting higher and higher glucose numbers. Of course, if you stopped training all together and just feeding yourself at the previous caloric amount, that glucose would be turned into fat and stored in your adipose (fat) tissues. For you as an athlete, when you see this occurring after a rest week, or two rest weeks, then this should be a signal to you that your glycogen stores are full, and you're ready to train again. A further confirmation is that within two days of restarting your intensive training, the levels come back to your previous norm. Figure 5.5 shows my glucose after I had 10 days of recovery after a two-week training camp. This shows that with a balanced meal of healthy vegetables, grains, and greens, my glucose rose to over 180 mg/d and stayed there until my late afternoon bike workout. Even though I don't have any signs of insulin resistance, this graph could be misinterpreted as showing a slow return to "post-meal baseline" and insulin resistance. This is why it is so important to understand the context in which you are interpreting your glucose curves. In this case, this slow return is actually just an indicator that my glycogen stores are full and I am recovered and ready for more training.

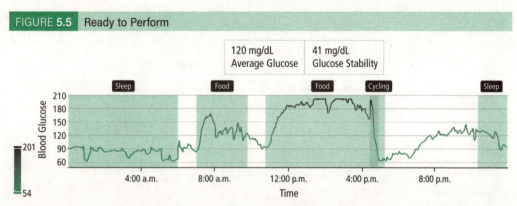

The tanks are full! When your glycogen stores are full, your blood glucose will be high and stay high after a meal. This is perfectly fine and a good indicator you're ready to perform.

How Do You Know That You Are Low in Your Glycogen Stores?

Let's consider the opposite scenario where you've been training hard, are tired, sore, and fatigued over multiple days. What happens with your blood glucose in this case? Your blood glucose does the opposite of the scenario above. For example, let's say your baseline is 90 mg/dL and you regularly cruise in life at this level. Your GPZ is between 110 and 145 mg/dL and when you feel like you're getting low in blood glucose, you notice your blood glucose at 75 mg/dL pretty consistently. Now, after three weeks of consistent and intense workouts or competitions, you find that your new baseline is 75 mg/dL, and that you don't feel hungry or low in blood glucose until around 60 mg/dL. "Wow, this is crazy!" you say. On the flip side, when you ingest carbs before and during training, it's very hard to raise your blood glucose to 110 mg/dL now, which was the low end previously. Even deliberately trying to spike it won't raise your blood glucose over 110 mg/dL. Not only that, but it feels like you're running on "fumes" during your training; you're constantly on the blood glucose roller coaster and struggling with workouts. This should be an indicator to you that it's time to rest and recover. See Figure 5.6. Sometimes, that's just not possible, especially if you're a professional cyclist competing in the Tour de France. In that case, you would need to eat and drink as many calories as possible consisting of carbs, proteins, and fats. You would need to stuff yourself for multiple days and see if you can restore some liver and muscle glycogen, otherwise it's going to be game over.

What Happens when You Start a Competition Hard from the Gun?

Have you ever watched those Olympic middle-distance runners? They start out fast and just get faster. There is no easing into the effort or ramping into the first lap. It's hard from the gun. There are many competitions where you have to be 100% prepared for maximal effort from the

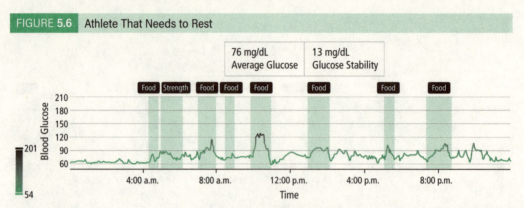

FIGURE 5.6 Athlete That Needs to Rest

New low baseline. This shows that no matter how much this athlete snacks or eats at meals, they're so depleted that they're not able to raise their blood glucose significantly. This athlete needs to rest and replenish their glycogen stores.

start. We talked about how to prepare yourself for this in the section on priming. What happens if you don't prime? In high pressure events like the Olympics, or an important event for you, or even just your first event where you might be anxious or nervous, your body will release adrenaline. This will also cause the liver to release glycogen (glycogenolysis) into circulation in anticipation of your effort.[55] This is a good thing. It's a natural priming and raising of blood glucose values to prepare you for the event. So, you should see an increase in your blood glucose 10 minutes or more before the event even starts. (The same thing can happen if you've to do a big presentation at work, for example. Remember: mood, movement, and food?) If you're a slow responder or someone that doesn't get too worked up by things, including competitions or workouts, then you'll not see a spike in glucose until about 5 to 15 minutes into the effort, and then you'll see this delayed spike. This is not ideal for an intense effort, hence the need for priming. See Figure 5.7.

What Does the Curve Look Like when Doing Maximal Exercise?

For many athletes, doing maximal exercise will cause a blood glucose spike and then continue to keep the blood glucose high throughout the effort (as long as it doesn't exceed two and a half hours, as it's unlikely you can maintain that high of a level for that long), which is a good thing and something that you want to create if possible. Yes, this is another time when you want a higher blood glucose level and, yes, it's perfectly healthy and fine for you to do this. You've been doing it all your life. Now that you have a CGM, you're learning what those numbers are. In Figure 5.8 we see an athlete doing an all-out 1-hour run for a PR in a 10-mile run event. Their blood glucose rises and stays pegged at the top end of their GPZ for the entire run. This is a great example of their body releasing a large amount of glucose to fuel their effort.

Now, don't worry if you can't get your blood glucose up during these kinds of efforts. There are some people with metabolisms that just don't respond in the same way. Also,

CHAPTER 5: Strategies on CGM Use for Performance   85

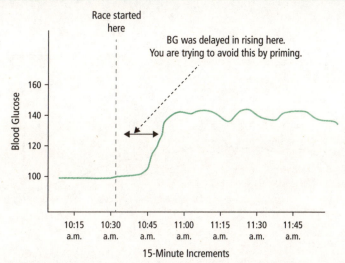

FIGURE 5.7 Competition Without Priming

Without priming, you could have a delayed rise in blood glucose that could put you behind your competitors in the beginning.

remember that 180+mg/dL isn't the goal, it's just what the athlete in Figure 5.8 could do. Maybe, for you, that's getting your blood glucose up to 125 mg/dL and then holding there. Remember from Chapter 1 that your glucose level is based on many things, and that basal level means your basal level. So, for you, a high level of blood glucose is 125 mg/dL. What's important in this scenario is that you *are* raising your blood glucose during maximal exercise.

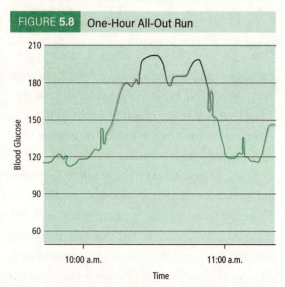

FIGURE 5.8 One-Hour All-Out Run

An appropriate glucose response for an athlete doing an all-out effort.

What Does It Mean If Your Glucose Drops During a Workout, and Continues to Drop?

This usually occurs when you're exercising for a longer period, longer than two and a half hours, so that you've used much of your liver glycogen and there is a reduction in circulating

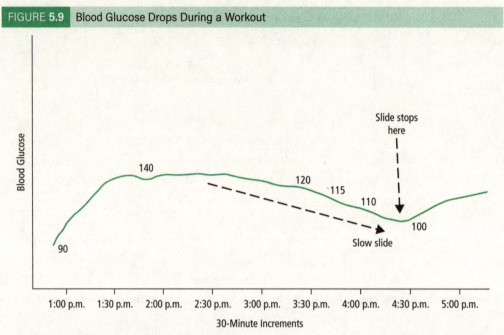

As previously mentioned in Chapter 4, the slow slide is an important pattern to recognize and stop before your glucose levels drop so much that it hinders your effort.

blood glucose, and you've also not ingested any carbs. This is hypoglycemia, which we have mentioned throughout the book, when you're low in blood sugar. How much drop is enough to make you feel hungry? How much is enough to make you feel "bonky?" Because everyone's basal level is different, the drop will be different, and it's largely dependent on what you're used to as your norm. If you're used to running at 130 mg/dL and you drop to 100 mg/dL, you'll feel like you need food immediately or you're going to bonk. Or if you're used to 80 mg/dL and then you drop to 65 mg/dL, you might feel bonky too. What are you concerned about from a performance standpoint? You want to minimize those drops, so that if you're on a slow slide from 130 to 100 mg/dL, you recognize it at 110 mg/dL and ingest more carbs (but not too much). See Figure 5.9, a clear example of the slow slide. This will help you to arrest that slide and stabilize your blood glucose at 110 mg/dL, and slowly bring it back up to 130 mg/dL in your optimal GPZ. Your job is to prevent the blood glucose from dropping too much while exercising. In Figure 5.10, we see a clear examples of a weightlifter who has low daily basal level, and even after eating a meal and then doing a run, his glucose levels remain very stable and lower than most people.

What Does It Mean If Your Glucose Never Comes up During Exercise and You've a Seemingly Abnormally Low Glucose Value?

Firstly, what is "normal?" Secondly, your sport might not demand a high level of blood glucose. In studying weightlifters and bodybuilders over the course of the past three years, I've found that all of them had a pretty low basal level and, during their workouts, they did not raise their blood glucose very high at all. Their daily average basal level was 80 mg/dL, and during hard lifting sessions, they would only raise their blood glucose to an average of 100 mg/dL. Weightlifting is based on muscular strength and the muscles don't need much circulating blood glucose. They rely more on the stored glycogen, therefore, their liver doesn't need to release much blood glucose into the bloodstream. Another reason is because you eat a low amount of carbohydrates. If you don't have the glucose, then it's not going to raise your blood glucose during exercise.

Lastly, you might just be in the small group of athletes that is almost a "non-responder" to glucose ingestion. Of course, there will be some response, but it might not be much, and it just appears that your glucose goes up 10–15 mg/dL and then right back to your baseline. That does happen in some people and that's just their unique metabolism. This could make it possibly challenging as an athlete though, especially if you're doing endurance sports. For sports that do not require a large amount of energy from glucose, then it's likely you will excel in those.

How Do You Find the Perfect Sports Drink or Gel for You?

Is there a perfect sports gel? How do you know which is right for you? Unfortunately, there's no simple answer or way to figure this out, except by testing them and seeing what happens. You're looking for three things from a glucose perspective.

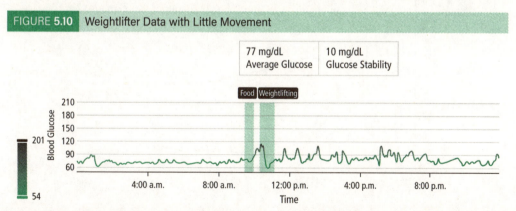

FIGURE 5.10 | Weightlifter Data with Little Movement

Weightlifting will not require a large change in glucose levels. If you have large muscle mass, the muscles act like a "storage house" for the glucose, so any glucose that you take in will be absorbed quickly.

1. It must contain a sugar that breaks down into glucose (glucose itself, dextrose, maltodextrin, or sucrose are preferred), and some fructose. Or it can be a "super-starch" like in the UCAN® products, so that you can get a rapid influx of glucose through your intestinal walls.
2. It needs to be at least 20 g of carbs.
3. It must give you a blood glucose spike, but not too much! This last one is the real trick and what you're testing for. You want your blood glucose to come up quickly, but not so quickly that your pancreas over secretes insulin and you create a reactive hypo crash. You want to ensure that your blood glucose comes up and stays up, again not too high.

Have a look at Figure 5.11, which shows two glucose curves. The taller curve is an example of too quickly and too tall of a glucose spike. The lower curve is more optimal and what you should strive for when ingesting fuel for a peak performance. This might take a little while to

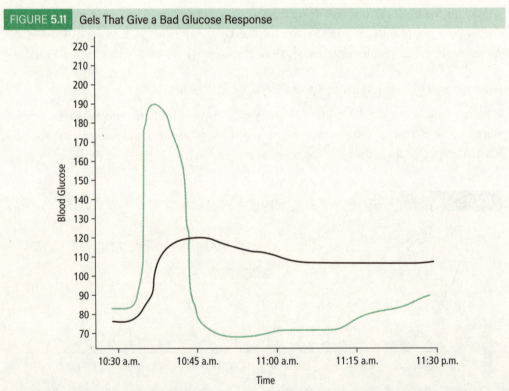

FIGURE 5.11 Gels That Give a Bad Glucose Response

One gel provides too quick of a large glucose spike with a hypo crash quickly following. Another gel provides a quick push up of glucose and no crash.

test. Buy a bunch of different gels and sports drinks, and start testing. Of course, you need to make it as repeatable as possible, so see if you can have the same meal before or always do it in the morning, etc. That's not always easy, but do your very best to make the conditions as close to the same as possible for your testing.

What Would a Keto Diet Look Like?

First off, a reminder that a keto diet is not the answer. It will be very, very difficult, if not impossible, to perform at a high level without carbohydrates. While it's true that you can do exercise on a low/no carb diet, it will have to be very low intensity. Once you reach around 70% of your maximum effort, your body will switch over to using mostly all carbs for fuel. So, a sport that is lower intensity can be done on keto, but only if you keep it low intensity. There are plenty of stories of endurance athletes out there that ride for 8 to 12 hours, or more, without carbs. They're burning fat and some muscle protein, and the body will produce its own glucose through glyconeogenesis to keep it going, but this is at a slow endurance pace. So, if you want to improve and push yourself to the next level, then you'll need carbs. Period. End of story.

What does a keto diet look like? It's a flat line. There is no blood glucose circulating, so the line will be down at 70 mg/dL or so and stay there the entire time. I know that when you first get your CGM and start to use it, you see those spikes and think: "Oh no, another spike, I need to eat less carbs and just eat protein and fats from now on." It's tempting to do it, but that's not the goal of creating a high-performing person, nor a healthy person. You need fiber, vegetables, complex carbs from grains, simple carbs from fruits, healthy lean proteins, and healthy unsaturated fats (no more seed oils!) to give your body the vitamins, minerals, antioxidants, and cancer-fighting nutrients to perform well and be healthy.

How Do I Know If I Did the Right Fueling?

We've talked about the right fueling already in Chapter 4 and about using your GPZs to keep your blood glucose within an optimal range for you. You've learned how to minimize your variability and keep your blood glucose more stable. You understand now how to prevent roller coasters during your workouts and reactive hypo and normal hypo crashes. The correct fueling means that you're eating something every 30 minutes or so, to keep the blood glucose up and stable and not letting it drop down over your entire workout or competition. Many athletes allow their blood glucose to drop and stay low, even a 15 mg/dL drop can impact your abilities, so it's super important to feed yourself throughout your workouts. This advice isn't new by any means, but now you can see the numbers on your CGM to help improve your performance. As Lord Kelvin said, "That which can be measured, can be improved."

How Do I Know If I Did the Wrong Fueling?

Generally, if you don't fuel correctly, you know it from your poor performance. However, many athletes never connect the dots between their poor performances and lack of fueling. I coached an elite female cyclist that had amazing numbers in training. Her testing was showing incredible improvements throughout the season, but she never performed well in races. She would always fade near the end and maybe come in 10th or 5th, but lacked that little bit extra to finish on the podium. We talked about hydration and nutrition and thought she was fueling correctly. It wasn't until I got a CGM on her in races that we saw she wasn't fueling as much as she thought she needed. She perceived that she was fine, but in reality her glucose went down dramatically at the end of her races. Only then did we both realize that she needed to take on way more carbs, in both liquid and solid form, throughout her races (and start much earlier in the races) so that when the last hour came around, she was "topped" off and able to race much harder. Instead of drinking only 30 g of carbs in her sports drink, we upped this to 60 g of carbs per hour, and then included two gels per hour, and every other hour a bar with it. By using the CGM and having her data available on her bike computer while racing, she could prevent a "slow slide" in the last hour as well. It was a game changer for her, and she began winning races right away.

There are many reasons for disappointing performances, from poor strategies or tactics to lack of concentration, dehydration, lack of fitness, heat and humidity, and the list goes on and on. One on the list is nutrition, and clearly glucose levels are a critical factor. Examining your blood glucose levels throughout your competition is a key place to observe whether you did indeed fuel correctly, often enough, and enough overall to excel. Keeping in your GPZs is very helpful, but it's not the end of the world if you slip out of them here and there. More concerning is a "roller coaster" throughout the competition, a slow slide, and a reactive hypoglycemic crash. If any of these three things appear in your post-competition data, then you'll know right away that, that could have been one of the reasons for your underachievement.

What If My Glucose Response Is Crazy Fast? Is There Such Thing As a "Hyper Sensitive" Responder?

As you know by now, there are many different responses, and those responses can change day to day, meal to meal, and certainly from person to person. So, yes, you could be faster than the fast responders mentioned in Chapter 3. Any little amount of glucose in your blood can spike you. This is not an issue *as long as* you also come back down. If you get a quick spike from a relatively small amount of glucose *and* stay up for a longer time (one hour or more) then you might have some signs of insulin resistance. How will this impact you as an athlete? You'll need to be more careful when you ingest simple carbs, and should consider a complex carb drink and foods, so that you have a slower reaction. I would also recommend that you include some healthy plant protein or protein powder in your sports drink, when you ingest carbs, to help slow down the blood glucose spike. The caveat to this is that when you're low in blood glucose because of multiple hard days of working out, or you've just completed an epic 24-hour race and now you are running on fumes, it would be "normal" to have a quick spike in response to a recovery shake or carb-heavy meal. In this case, the blood glucose will reduce quickly as it's getting soaked up by the cells as fast as they can pull it in.

My Baseline Glucose Used To Be 109 mg/dL, but Now It's 85 mg/dL After I've Improved My Fitness and Changed My Diet. Is That Okay? What Does That Mean?

A change in your basal glucose from a higher to lower glucose level is a good thing in most cases. I call this a glucose reset. This can occur over time, and it could take months of training and/or a change in diet to see this change. What this means is that you're now more insulin sensitive and your metabolism is working more efficiently. Most likely you've also lost some body fat, both in your adipose tissues (the stuff you see in the mirror!) and internally around your organs, and even intra-cellularly. These have all created a greater sensitivity of your cells to insulin (more efficient and effective), so that you need less and less insulin to reduce your blood glucose levels, and the glucose you're taking in fills the cell receptors instead of fats (more on this in Chapter 8).

This glucose reset is a good thing and should be celebrated (just not with a jelly dough-nut!). I have seen this occur in multiple athletes now, both in an improved fitness level and weight loss, and in a change in diet. A change from an omnivore diet to a whole foods plant-based diet can cause a drop in your baseline after some time (it might take six months). This diet can make a big difference in your average daily glucose levels, as you substitute animal proteins for plants with antioxidants, tons of fiber, healthy complex carbs, and proteins. As an athlete, it's something to consider especially if your basal blood glucose is over 100 mg/dL on average per day. This can also occur in the opposite (wrong) direction as well, if you're not being careful with your nutrition and have stopped exercising at your previous level. If your blood glucose goes from 95 to 120 mg/dL over time, say six months, then you need to mend your evil ways! Clean up your nutrition and start exercising on a regular basis again.

What are the caveats to this one? You could think that you're experiencing a glucose reset if your blood glucose goes up, but actually it's just a short period of time during a rest and/or taper week as you prepare for a peak of fitness. See Figure 5.12. In this case, know that as soon as you start training/competing again, your blood glucose will return to its previous basal level. On the flip side, we've talked about how you can experience a temporary glucose reset at the

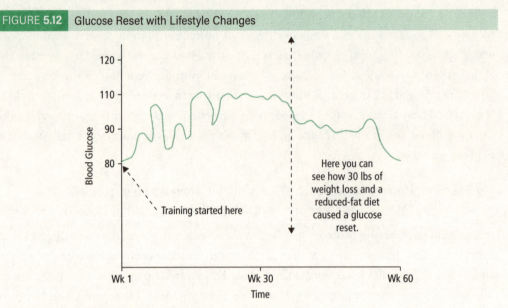

A glucose reset can occur after an increase in fitness or a change in diet.

end of a hard training cycle. In this case, if you still have another week or more to train, then you do need to readjust your brain to the new lower levels, and see if you can begin to ingest more carbs each day to begin replenishing your muscle glycogen stores.

The key to understanding your blood glucose is watching it carefully over a period of at least six months. It's difficult to go through enough different life and athletic scenarios in less time to fully understand all the different responses, your baseline, and your reactions when fatigued and when rested, etc. Eventually you'll put together a "library" in your head of your responses, and you'll know what caused them, what will happen next, and even be in control of your blood glucose for nearly every situation, whether that's life, working out, or competing.

CHAPTER 6

Learn From Others' Data

AMID ALL OF THIS SCIENCE, sometimes it's helpful to explain things using real-world examples, so that you can better understand your responses and how to improve your performance. These case studies are from athletes I've worked with over the past three years. They provide unique insights into their individual glucose responses, which I've seen not only in these athletes but in many others. So while that could be considered a trend, I also know that many factors are involved. As you read these, remember that the "lowest" quality of science is anecdotes. Still, I do believe it's essential to read about others' experiences, as many times you'll find something that resonates with your experience, and you'll gain practical advice from this. I've selected these case studies because I've seen them occur over and over. I've also included examples of athletes making mistakes, so you can avoid them.

A WEEK OF HARD TRAINING

Joe Athlete is a 42-year-old male cyclist who has been training for a week-long cycling trip. See Figure 6.0. He'll ride for four to six hours each day on rolling and mountainous terrain. With the length and intensity of this cycling, he'll burn an additional 2500–3000 kilocalories (k/cals) per day over his normal metabolic rate of roughly 2500 k/cals.

Leading into the week-long trip, he took an easier week to ensure his muscles were recovered, glycogen stores were full, and he had plenty of energy to be ready to tackle the 7-day trip. His fasted, morning glucose level is between 90–95 mg/dL, and his pre-meal baseline is 100–110 mg/dL. By reducing his workload in the week before the cycling trip, he recovered both from a cardiac and muscular standpoint. At the end of this easy/rest week, his fasted, morning glucose level raised to 100–106 mg/dL and his pre-meal baseline raised to 110–120 mg/dL. This could indicate that the muscle and liver glycogen stores are full, and while we can't definitively say that's true, from a scientific standpoint it's highly likely this is the case. He stated, "At the end of my rest week, I felt like I was going to jump out of my skin. My legs were twitching and ready to go!" One might also consider that during a rest week,

93

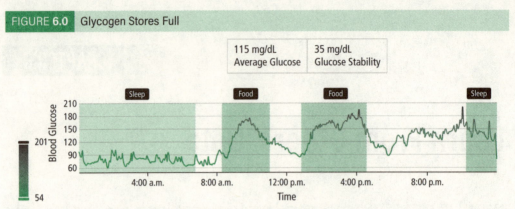

Joe Athlete's increase in fasting glucose after a rest week resulted in a 10 mg/dL rise from his normal training week. This could indicate that his glycogen stores are full in his muscles and liver.

training volume is reduced but food intake remains the same, which could be another reason fasting glucose is higher. Another possible explanation is that Joe has some insulin resistance going on, as we know that you can reverse type 2 diabetes through exercise (you'll learn more about this in the next chapter). So, during training, he has no insulin resistance, but when he rests, it returns. It's difficult to say which is correct as no one has studied this exact scenario yet, of an increase in fasting glucose at the end of a rest week.[56]

At the start of his cycling trip, his glucose levels stayed higher than usual, by 10–20 mg/dL for the first two days, and on the third day, his levels came down to his "usual" pre-meal baseline. By day seven, he was highly fatigued and now his glucose levels were much lower. He was riding at an 80–90 mg/dL level, with a morning fasted glucose of 70. Clearly, he now has a new baseline, as he has depleted his glycogen stores daily, and it's likely he's not taken in enough glucose after his rides to replenish those stores completely.[57] Every bite of carbs will fuel his current activities, and any extra will replenish his muscle glycogen stores, but there's not enough glucose or time to do this before the next ride. However, he doesn't necessarily feel like he has low glucose, and has no symptoms of hypoglycemia either, and he finished day seven with the front group and feeling strong. His body is now getting "used to" a lower level of glucose and this is his new pre-meal baseline. See Figure 6.1.

This is a common occurrence after a hard week, or even longer, of training. It should also be noted that if you see your fasted glucose dropping during a week-long type training or competition, you might also consider that you're not putting enough carbohydrates back in to replenish your stores. Using a continuous glucose monitor (CGM) to help direct your carbohydrate and overall caloric intake is a great way to ensure that you're recovering optimally for the following workout or event.

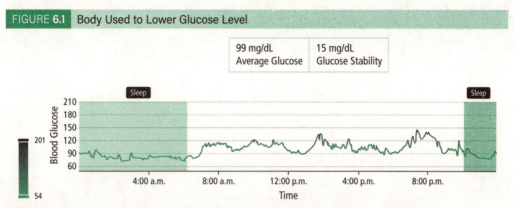

Joe Athlete's new pre-meal baseline is 30 mg/dL lower than before the week-long cycling trip. He's not exhibiting any hypoglycemic symptoms, which means his body has gotten used to the new lower level of glucose.

REACTIVE HYPOGLYCEMIC CRASH

Jill CrossFitter has been doing CrossFit now for two years and loves the camaraderie, the support, and her workout "family." She has been struggling lately with keeping her energy high toward the end of her workouts, and she feels like this is because of a lack of nutrition. So she bought a CGM and started wearing it to see if she could learn something about her glucose before, during, and after her workouts. The first thing she learned was that she had a fasting glucose level of 75 mg/dL and her pre-meal glucose baseline was 85 mg/dL. She works out early in the morning before work and normally gets up, grabs some black coffee and heads to the CrossFit gym. She noticed that after the coffee and movement in the morning, her glucose comes up to 85–90 mg/dL, but then stabilizes and stays there for the first 20 minutes of her workout. She then sees that it drops to 75 mg/dL, and it continues dropping, heading down to 60 mg/dL in the last 10 minutes of the workout. That's too low! For sure, this is a hypoglycemic state, and she decided that she should try some sports gels before her workouts. She bought some and then took two on the 20-minute drive from her home to the CrossFit gym. A tasty, sweet, chocolate treat, she thought, and surely this would help her to increase her glucose levels.

She got to the gym and noticed right before the workout, her glucose had risen to 145 mg/dL—clearly those gels had an impact. About 45 minutes in, she had a big, rapid drop in her glucose, from 130 mg/dL to 60 mg/dL, and she didn't think she was going to be able to finish the last 15 minutes. She got shaky, a little dizzy, and had to sit down, rest, and drink some cold water. She couldn't understand what was happening. What had happened? She had a reactive hypoglycemic crash to the two gels she ingested. See Figure 6.2. By raising her glucose so quickly and high, her pancreas released insulin to deal with that glucose while she was still "at

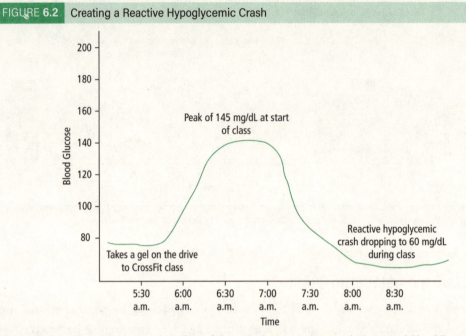

FIGURE 6.2 Creating a Reactive Hypoglycemic Crash

Jill Crossfitter creates a reactive hypoglycemic crash because she ingested too much glucose quickly while at rest, and then didn't follow it up with additional glucose to help keep her level high for her workout.

rest" while driving to class. When she began working out and exercising, her muscle cells, which are highly sensitive to taking up glucose,[58] began moving the glucose out of the bloodstream. This, combined with a release of insulin, led her body to clear the circulating glucose so quickly (it still took 45 minutes, so not that fast) that she became hypoglycemic. To be clear, Jill "created" the reactive hypoglycemic crash, and I've found that this is a common occurrence among many athletes, and they don't even know they're doing it to themselves. Reminder: A reactive hypoglycemic crash is characterized by a lower glucose level than you had before the ingestion of carbs.

The next day, she decided to take one gel 30 minutes into her workout, instead of taking two gels before her workout, to see what would happen. See Figure 6.3. At the time, her glucose had dropped to 70 mg/dL. After taking the gel, within 10 minutes, her glucose was trending upward and had risen to 85 mg/dL, and she finished the workout with a glucose of 100 mg/dL feeling strong. What was the difference? She took the gel during exercise. When you're exercising, your body doesn't release much, if any, insulin, as your muscles are so receptive to the glucose that they absorb it quickly. Therefore, this time, she didn't have the combination

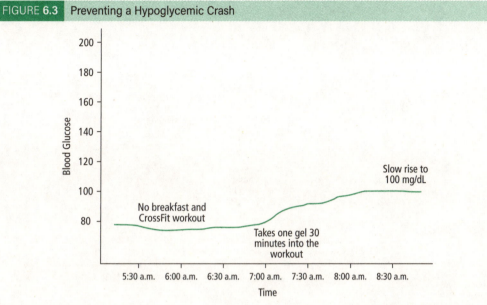

Jill Crossfitter takes a gel 30 minutes into her workout, which helps to raise her glucose levels but does not cause a reactive hypoglycemic crash.

of insulin *and* muscle uptake (during exercise) working together to reduce the circulating glucose.

Jill loves using her new CGM and decides to do another experiment on herself on the third workout of the week. This time, she takes the two gels in the car on the way to CrossFit, but she also has two more in her pocket to anticipate the reactive hypoglycemic crash. See Figure 6.4. She watches her glucose go from 75 mg/dL to 145 mg/dL again. Ten minutes after beginning her workout, she notices that the trend arrow is pointing straight down, as her glucose is now 125 mg/dL. She takes another gel immediately, continues with her exercises, and then 10 minutes later looks again at her CGM app and sees that she's still trending downward, but not as quickly and is now at 115 mg/dL. She takes another gel now, and within 10 minutes her glucose has risen to 130 mg/dL, and she finishes her workout stronger than ever before.

Jill has learned that she can prevent a low glucose situation with sports gels. By taking sports gels during her workout, or both pre-workout and during her workout, she can enhance her performance. She will need to decide which protocol she wants to continue to do in the future, but both work.

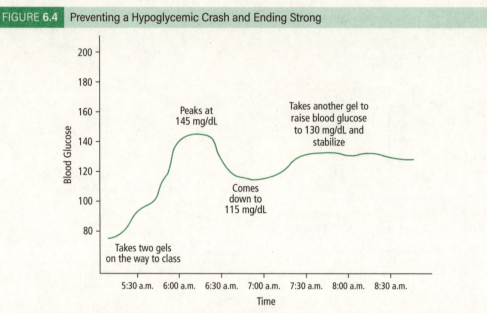

FIGURE 6.4 Preventing a Hypoglycemic Crash and Ending Strong

Jill Crossfitter takes two gels in the car on the way to class, takes another 10 minutes into class, and another one 20 minutes into class. She maintains a higher level of glucose all the way to the end of class and also avoids a reactive hypoglycemic crash.

WEIGHTLIFTER WITH EXCELLENT GLUCOSE TOLERANCE

Jeff Weightlifter has been lifting weights for about five years, and is lean and muscular, weighing 245 lbs and standing at 5' 10" tall. He is now 30 and has just gotten a CGM to see how he can ensure he doesn't have any insulin resistance. He wants to improve his overall longevity and vitality and, of course, his workouts. Jeff's fasting glucose is 95 mg/dL and pre-meal glucose is 105 mg/dL. After two weeks on the sensor, he sees that his glucose stays pretty stable all the time and he very rarely has big spikes. He eats healthily, with plenty of vegetables, legumes, and good, low-in-saturated-fat meats, and is serious about getting better and better in the weight room, with an eye toward doing a weightlifting contest in the next six months. See Figure 6.5.

Jeff decided to try to increase his glucose for his workouts, to see if that would give him extra energy and help him lift even harder. Jeff bought an energy drink loaded in caffeine and sugar, and once his workout started, he opened it and drank it down. At the beginning of the workout, his glucose was 110 mg/dL, and throughout the workout his glucose barely came up, but did rise to 125 mg/dL by the end. Jeff was surprised that his glucose didn't go any higher; however, he did have a good workout and felt strong at the end. So, he decided at his next workout he was going

CHAPTER 6: Learn From Others' Data

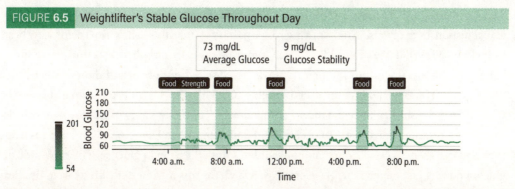

FIGURE 6.5 Weightlifter's Stable Glucose Throughout Day

Jeff Weightlifter with a usual day of glucose values. He has a very stable glucose level all day long, with small spikes from his meals and snacks.

to have an energy drink and two sports gels to see if that would raise his glucose. The same thing happened: he just didn't have much increase in glucose, and this time his glucose rose to the same 125 mg/dL-level despite including an additional 40 g of high-glycemic carbs. For his third workout, he went all out. He had the energy drink, a sports gel, and a candy bar. This time it was enough to move his glucose to 135 mg/dL, but still not a large spike. His workout went well, and he had plenty of energy, but nothing special. He decided that while the energy drink helped him with focus, he didn't really feel any different from the gels or candy bar.

What could be going on with Jeff? Firstly, he doesn't have to worry about any insulin resistance as his glucose is very stable. It barely rises with a fairly large increase in glucose, and clearly, he has good glucose tolerance. Secondly, Jeff has a lot of muscle mass. Muscles soak up glucose. Jeff has so much muscle mass that he likely can handle a lot more glucose than most people before experiencing a glucose spike. Maybe he just needs to take in a lot more glucose to cause a spike? Certainly, a possibility. Lastly, we need to consider the effects of the caffeine in his energy drink. Most energy drinks have between 70 and 125 mg of caffeine. Caffeine improves absorption of carbohydrates but at much higher levels than Jeff ingested (5 mg/kg/hr).[59] Combined with glucose, caffeine does increase the rate of carbohydrate oxidation (burning/usage). It's been shown that you can increase your carbohydrate burn by 26% during the final 30 minutes of exercise over the ingestion of glucose alone.[60]

TRIATHLETE WITH HYPER RESPONDER TO GLUCOSE INGESTION

Julie Triathlete has been a competitive age-group triathlete now for eight years, and she's qualified for the big Ironman in Hawaii, which she believes she can place in the top five if all goes well. She's 43 years old, trains roughly 15 to 20 hours a week, and is very focused on improving.

She's been using a CGM for two months and is just starting to understand more about her individual responses to glucose. She's starting to see patterns, and thinks she's also seeing how best to fuel herself. What she's found is that any time she takes in carbohydrates during training, her glucose shoots up to 160–180 mg/dL, stays there for an hour or so, and then slowly comes down. She's able to watch it come down roughly 10–15 mg/dL at a time, and when she sees it reach 115 mg/dL, she begins to eat more carbohydrates. This "slow slide" of glucose over time is a super important characteristic to observe and understand. See Figure 6.6. This happens over time and can seem to be so slow that many athletes miss the drop in glucose. The slow slide of glucose doesn't just happen during exercise, so watch for this in your daily life as well. Besides recognizing the drop in glucose, it's important to not overfeed and create a reactive hypoglycemic crash when there doesn't need to be one. During the slow slide, when she sees that 115 mg/dL mark, Julie takes in two gummy cubes and sucks on them for a few minutes, then chews and swallows them. She waits 5 to 10 minutes, and repeats if the first two did not stop the slow slide. Gummy cubes are an excellent way to slowly increase glucose without overdoing it. On the other hand, sometimes you do just need a bunch of carbs, and you need them now!

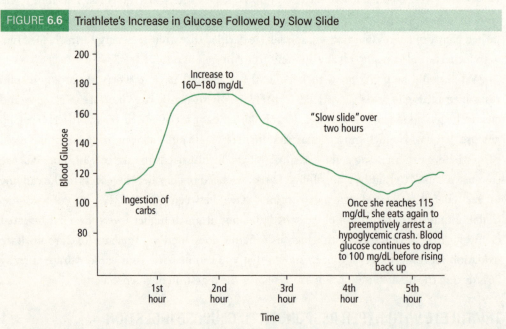

FIGURE 6.6 Triathlete's Increase in Glucose Followed by Slow Slide

Julie Triathlete has a large increase in glucose followed by a "slow slide." It's important to recognize the slow slide, and then determine when you need to arrest it and how many carbohydrates you should take to stop it.

What Julie also learned is that she has a very quick response to glucose intake. Nearly every day, Julie would have "naked" carbs, meaning carbs only, without any fiber, proteins, or fats. She would have an increase of glucose by 80–100 mg/dL, and it would happen within 10 minutes of ingestion. See Figure 6.7. Now, if she wasn't exercising, she also had a normal and quick reduction in glucose, as her body either stored it as glycogen or burned it, or even stored it as fat. The question is: Should she try to reduce the peak of her spikes, even though she has a quick return to pre-meal baseline? I would argue, yes. A reduction in the magnitude of the glucose peak is desirable and healthy. The science also says that reducing the magnitude of the glucose spikes is healthier for the endothelial cells that make up the inner cell walls in the vessels.[61] What Julie found was that by adding in some healthy fats, like ground flax, hemp hearts, nuts, or avocado to her carbs, or by adding in fiber with vegetables and salad, she could reduce the sheer peak of her spikes by nearly 40–50 mg/dL. See Figure 6.8. That's worth doing! Healthy protein will also help you to reduce those spikes, especially when combined with fibrous vegetables. You'll learn more about how to reduce your glucose spikes in Chapter 8.

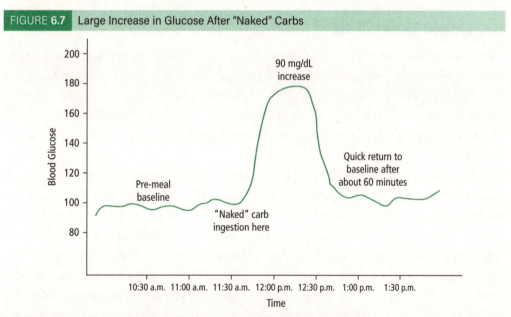

FIGURE 6.7 Large Increase in Glucose After "Naked" Carbs

Julie has a very quick and large increase in glucose when she has "naked" carbs.

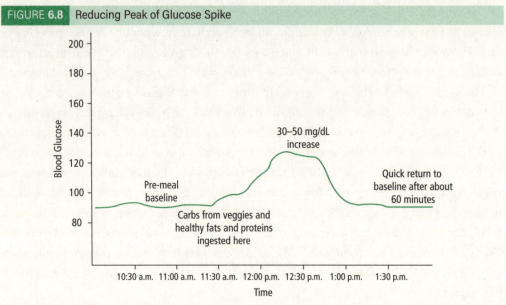

FIGURE 6.8 Reducing Peak of Glucose Spike

By adding in some fiber (vegetables), healthy fats, and protein, Julie is able to reduce the peak of the glucose spike by 40–50 mg/dL.

WHAT ABOUT THE KETO DIET?

The keto/paleo/carnivore diets are all lumped into one category. They're not the same diets, but do have a major commonality between them: they're high protein and high fat. These diets typically will have over 90% of their calories from protein and fats, and some strict adherents to them will consume no carbohydrates. There are many people who follow this nutritional diet and praise it highly for having helped them lose weight and improve their health.

How well does this work for athletes? It can work if you're doing a sport that doesn't require high intensity. So, keeping your intensity under 70% of your threshold heart rate allows you to continue to burn fats, and not have to use a higher percentage of your glycogen stores. (There is no "on/off" switch in the body determining to burn fat or carbs. It's more of a percentage, where one is oxidized more than the other.) Because these athletes don't consume carbohydrates, it's nearly impossible for them to train and/or compete at a high level of intensity. They *can* do it, but only until their limited glycogen stores are depleted, so roughly one and a half hours. Remember that the body can produce its own glucose through the process of gluconeogenesis, but this is a slow process and certainly can't keep up with high-intensity exercise. While there have been entire books written about each of these diets and how great they are, one thing is true for athletes: it's not for you! If you're doing any kind of high-intensity training or competition, you need carbs. You must have a large storage of muscle and liver glycogen, and then plenty of circulating glucose molecules to provide you with enough energy to train and compete at a high level.

Bob Cyclist decided to try out the carnivore diet to see if he could lose some stubborn weight and to see if he could continue to train in cycling at the same intensity as he does when on a more varied diet. See Figure 6.9. Bob immediately began losing some weight, as he had decreased his overall caloric intake (one side benefit of animal protein is the feeling of satiety it gives you) and he continued to exercise between 8 and 10 hours a week. After hearing about CGMs, he became curious and wondered what was happening with his glucose levels while on the carnivore diet, and during exercise. He immediately found that his glucose levels were very stable, and he had no real spikes. That makes perfect sense, he wasn't ingesting any carbs! During exercise, he found it was tough to ride longer than three hours. However, as long as he kept his pace low, and under roughly 70% of his threshold heart rate, he was able to make three hours, and up to four and a half hours, which was as long as he wanted to ride anyhow. Recovery definitely was not the same though, and he found it took at least two days longer than his normal recovery time if he had done a long, steady distance ride. This also makes sense, as there are hundreds of studies proving the importance of carbohydrates in recovery post-exercise.[62] While Bob could certainly exercise, there was a limit to intensity and recovery. In the end, Bob stuck with it for about seven months, lost 40 lbs of

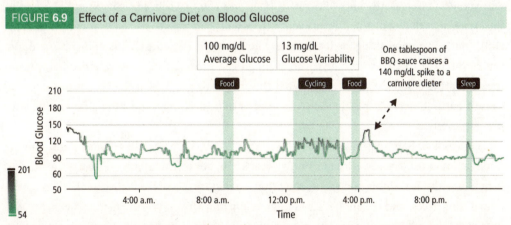

FIGURE 6.9 Effect of a Carnivore Diet on Blood Glucose

Bob Cyclist on a carnivore diet maintains nearly a flat line of glucose all day as there isn't any ingestion of glucose to raise the levels.

weight, and then went back to a more balanced diet, which allowed him to increase his intensity on the bike and keep the weight off. I would be remiss if I also didn't mention the potential negative health consequences of this kind of diet. Animal protein has been correlated with colon, prostate, and breast cancer, among others,[63] and the lack of fiber makes it tough (pun intended) to pass food through the digestive tract. A diet rich in animal protein lacks in antioxidants that are highly protective in your body, and it's unknown whether this kind of diet is good for your cardiovascular health. There is only one long-term study (five years) looking at cardiovascular health indicators and high animal protein diet, and it actually found the participants had no different levels of occluded arteries than those on a "normal" diet that contained vegetables, fruits, and animal proteins.[64] For certain, more research needs to be done in this area.

POOR FUELING STRATEGY, A BAD RESULT IN AN EVENT, AND THE IMPACT OF ADRENALIN

One of the exciting things about using a CGM is that you can do some experimenting on yourself, to see how you react to different fueling strategies, determine which one works best for you, and then move forward with that strategy for future training and events. You should always do your testing during training, as you don't want to waste a great race because you were trying out something new in your nutrition routine. With this strategy, you can determine the best types of pre-event meal to give you the glucose level you want before your event, then understand how best to fuel during your event, and finally, learn what to do after your event for optimal recovery. The unknown in trying a new strategy with regards to glucose is that you don't necessarily know how your body will react to the "pre-race jitters." Normally, the excitement that comes before an event causes your pancreas to release epinephrine (adrenalin), which is a good thing, as it prepares your body for the effort. This epinephrine dump causes the liver to free stored glycogen through the process of glycogenolysism, and raises the circulating blood glucose levels.[65] What this means to you, is that the pre-event jitters can cause a natural increase in glucose, so this needs to be accounted for as you determine your pre-event nutrition.

Let's look at Ralph Racer. Ralph is a bike racer, 25 years old, who has come up through the ranks and is considered an elite racer now—not a pro, but top amateur. He's gotten a CGM to help him with his training and racing nutrition, so that he can prevent the "bonk" (hypoglycemia) during races, and ensure he has enough energy for the end of the races, where the winners make the winning moves. The morning of a big event, he has a pancake breakfast with syrup, and some eggs and sausage. The pancakes with syrup are high glycemic, and even with some protein and fat to slow down his absorption of that glucose, it increases his glucose from

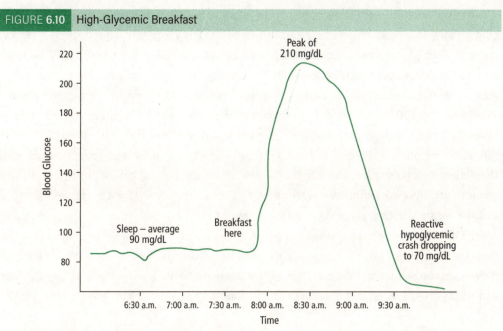

Ralph's breakfast with high-glycemic foods creates a large spike in glucose and then a reactive hypoglycemic crash.

his fasted glucose of 90 mg/dL to 210 mg/dL. That's a huge increase, especially for someone without any other signs of insulin resistance, and goes to show just how much of an increase can occur if you ingest a ton of simple sugars at breakfast. See Figure 6.10.

Now you can imagine what happens next, right? His pancreas releases too much insulin, drives all that glucose into his cells very rapidly, and he has a reactive hypoglycemic crash an hour later, which is only an hour before the start of his race. He doesn't recognize it at first, as he's busy at the race site preparing to race, but then starts to feel sluggish and a bit dizzy. He looks at his CGM app and sees he's down to 70 mg/dL, and then puts two and two together. He stops what he's doing and has a sports bar and apple slices with almond butter to help bring his glucose back up, and hopefully stabilize it. His glucose indeed comes back up to 100 mg/dL, and rises further to 120 mg/dL, with the trend arrow pointing diagonally upward and at the right time, as it's 15 minutes before the start. Now, with five minutes to the start, he looks at his glucose on his bicycle computer and sees it's 150 mg/dL, as he's quite excited for the race and his pancreas has released glucagon because of the epinephrine dump that's occurring. That glucagon is telling the liver to release a bunch of glucose from the glycogen stores into the bloodstream. "We have a race starting soon and are going to need energy here people!" Once the race starts, Ralph watches his glucose levels closely, as he knows it's going to be a hard race.

Within 15 minutes of the start, he sees his glucose back down to 115 mg/dL, and it's dropping rapidly, so he eats a sports bar and drinks half of his sports drink for a total of 60 g of carbs. Within 10 minutes, his glucose stops dropping and stabilizes at 135 mg/dL, which is right in his glucose performance zone (GPZ) for racing. As he gets caught up in racing, he forgets to eat, and after an hour he notices that he's been on a slow slide for the past hour, and is back down to 100 mg/dL, and feeling pretty tired. He takes all eight gummy blocks in his pocket, stuffs them in his mouth and chews them down. He needs a boost quickly, which this works for, but it works too well and within 15 minutes, he's now at 200 mg/dL. In another 15 minutes, he's having a reactive hypoglycemic crash and he's back down to 85 mg/dL, and about to get dropped. Unfortunately for him, this is exactly when the race winner is decided, and the racing becomes particularly difficult, and he gets dropped from the group as he just doesn't have the power to keep up at this point. Here's a perfect example of fueling improperly, from the time he got up in the morning to when he got dropped out of the group in the race. Relying on too many simple sugars, not paying attention to his glucose levels during the race, and then over-ingesting gummy blocks all contributed to a poor result. See Figure 6.11. This

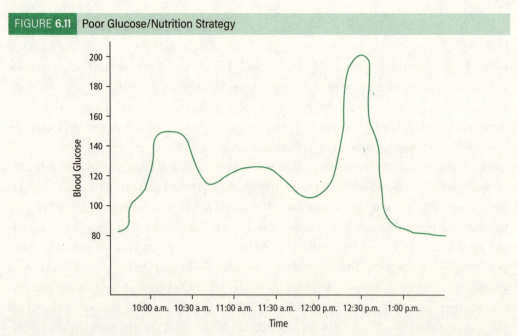

FIGURE 6.11 Poor Glucose/Nutrition Strategy

Ralph's race doesn't go as planned due to a poor nutritional strategy. He doesn't keep his glucose levels high enough, discovers this too late, and then overfeeds simple sugars, which causes another reactive hypoglycemic crash, and he gets dropped from the small winning group of racers.

CHAPTER 6: Learn From Others' Data   107

poor result comes purely from a poor nutrition strategy, and not from the lack of ability to be with the winning riders. It's a scenario that plays out all too often in many sports competitions, not just cycling.

PERFECT FUELING AND A GREAT RACE RESULT

On the positive side, we have Michelle Beltran, who is a 54-year-old former professional cyclist, and now has come back to the sport of cycling, and is out to dominate all the world's toughest gravel cycling races. Gravel racing is a bicycle race done on gravel roads, and is usually quite long, upward of 10 hours. I've coached Michelle for over two years, and we've been fortunate to use a Supersapiens CGM for quite a while to learn the best way to plan her glucose strategy. Michelle's main goal for the season is a 200-mile race through the gravel roads of Kansas, called Unbound. She wants to win her age group, and has been training extensively for the event. Using her CGM in training, she's learned that as long as she eats or drinks some carbs every 30 minutes through the race, and even eats something more substantial with protein and fats in it, like a protein bar or sandwich, then she'll be able to keep her glucose between 90 mg/dL and 150 mg/dL, which is where she has found her best performances.

Michelle's fasting glucose is 90 mg/dL, and she starts out with a breakfast of her own concoction of cereal that contains ground flaxseeds, muesli, hemp hearts, and Ezekiel cereal, with two tablespoons of almond butter and unsweetened organic soy milk. She has found that this will give her a glucose boost, but not too much, and sustains her energy for most of the morning. Waking up at 4:00 a.m. for a 6:30 a.m. race start, which is not the normal routine for her, along with the dump of epinephrine that comes from being excited about the race, causes her glucose to rise higher with a brief blip at 150 mg/dL, a correction, and then stabilizing at 120 mg/dL right before the race start.

Once the race starts, her glucose shoots up to 190 mg/dL without any additional ingestion of glucose, as she's highly responsive to another big dump of epinephrine in the first part of the race. This does not frazzle her, as she's seen it before and knows to just stick with her schedule of eating every 30 minutes. If she does that, she'll be able to sustain her energy levels. After an hour of racing, she begins the slow slide of glucose, and slowly drops down to 90 mg/dL over the next two hours. She continues to eat every 30 minutes, watching her glucose on her bike computer. When she drops below 120 mg/dL, she eats double what she has been normally eating to ensure she doesn't drop too far. After bottoming out at 90 mg/dL, her glucose comes up to 110–115 mg/dL and stays there over two more hours. She drops one more time around 1:00 p.m. and eats a sandwich of almond butter and jam, with a small bag of chips, a sports bar, and two bottles of sports drink. This big meal causes her glucose

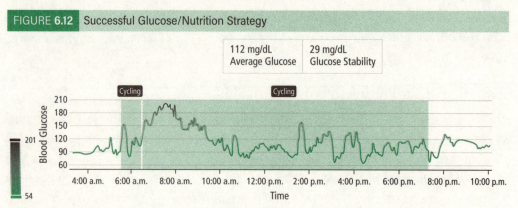

A very successful glucose/nutrition strategy in the 200-mile unbound gravel bike race, results in an age-group win by over two hours.

to rise to 155 mg/dL, but it quickly comes back down again and begins a slower rise to 130 mg/dL. This coincided with a big effort, so that was perfect timing to have her food. She used all those carbs and had a big drop in glucose at 3:00 p.m., but took in a sugary soda drink with 35 g of carbs, and had two gels which had 20 g each, so a total of 75 g of carbs, bringing her glucose back to nearly 150 mg/dL. However, this was a little too much at this point, and it's easy to see in Figure 6.12 that she had a bit of a reactive hypoglycemic crash dropping down to 60 mg/dL.

She makes another stop for fuel, and eats some sugary bacon for both the fat and sugar content, more pretzels, and a protein bar, and then has stable glucose for the next three and a half hours. The addition of protein at this point halted the "roller coaster" she was on. Normally, once you're on the roller coaster of high and low glucose, it's very hard to get off it. Generally, the only way to get off the roller coaster is to stop and eat some slow-digesting carbs with protein, so that your body doesn't have just a large load of high-glycemic carbs on board. Since she has done this to herself in training, and we've worked together for a long time, we've learned exactly what she needs to stop the roller coaster. The most critical thing in a racing situation is to have the availability of the food you need to stop the roller coaster. Otherwise, you just need to stay on, and keep feeding carbs to the finish. She has one final drop in glucose, at about 7:30 p.m., but takes in a gel, and then 20 minutes later takes in another one, followed by one more 20 minutes after that, for a total of 60 g in one hour. This is perfect pacing of carbs at this point, and brings her glucose up to 120, and she keeps it there until the finish of the race. Michelle wins her age category by over two hours to the second-place rider. Incredible fitness, and a clear understanding of glucose changes with a great nutrition strategy, resulted in a dominating performance.

NOT EATING ENOUGH AFTER A HARD WORKOUT TO RECOVER FOR THE NEXT DAY'S WORKOUT

This is one of the many lessons I learned in the past three years using a CGM and analyzing my own data. I coach 6 to 10 cycling camps a year, and one of my favorites is the gravel cycling camp held in the blue ridge mountains of Virginia. We ride some epic gravel roads with big climbs and descents, and end up with 4 to 7 hours of hard riding each day. A combined total of six days of hard riding, and using all my glycogen stores daily, means that eating enough afterward is critical for the following day's ride. Eating out at the local Mexican restaurant after our longest ride of the week (7 to 8 hours) is something that I always enjoy.

On "long day," I burned over 3600 k/cals, in addition to the estimated basal metabolic rate of 2400 k/cals. In 2022, I didn't eat enough at dinner, went to bed hungry, woke up at 1:30 a.m. starving, and looked at my glucose and saw I was down to 70 mg/dL, which is very low for me at night, as I generally average between 90 and 100 mg/dL. The next day I struggled to keep with the rest of the campers (not good if you're the coach!), had sore legs, and generally felt low in power with "empty" legs. Clearly, underfeeding at dinner made a major difference in my ability to perform the next day. My glycogen stores in my muscles must not have replenished. A big mistake!

In Figure 6.13, you can see that even though I had carbs for dinner, my glucose barely increased, as all my muscle cells were just soaking up everything I gave them. This was a great reminder of how important it is to have plenty of food for dinner after many hard days of riding. Instead of just eating a normal portion, I should have "stuffed" myself, leaving the restaurant with the feeling of an over-stuffed belly. While not comfortable, it would have been the

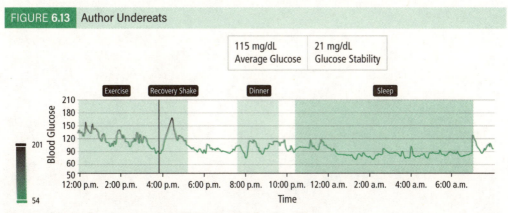

FIGURE 6.13   Author Undereats

Hunter undereats after a long day of coaching at his gravel cycling camp.

right thing to do. Or, I could have made myself another recovery shake after dinner to take in an additional 600–1000 k/cals before bed. Lesson learned.

These are just a few of the case studies that could be written about, as there are so many different scenarios and situations in which having a glucose strategy could be helpful. Understanding your individual response is critical to putting your CGM to use. It's important to remind you that there are many factors that influence your response, from the meal you had before your current meal, to your training status, to your mood, and even an injury or illness. It remains important that you be very observant of your own data, noting what foods and sports nutrition give you certain responses, and also that you experiment with new nutrition strategies. This can help you to learn even more about yourself.

CHAPTER 7

Diabetes and Athletic Performance: Using a CGM

"DURING EXERCISE, EVERYBODY HAS DIABETES!" says Phil Southerland, type 1 former pro cyclist, and founder of Team Type 1 and Supersapiens continuous glucose monitor (CGM) app. Phil Southerland arguably has *the* largest CGM data set of any type 1 athlete in the world. He started using a CGM in 1999, when he was a pro cyclist, and it was surgically placed under his skin at the top of his back. "I did my race weekend and then the next week, went to the doctor to download the data from the sensor in my back. I was blown away. I started the race at 90 mg/dL but within 10 minutes into the race, it was 330 mg/dL!"

Type 1 diabetes is a completely different scenario than type 2 diabetes, where the body produces insulin, but due to the presence of insulin resistance, insulin is not capable of fulfilling its role anymore. Athletes with type 1 diabetes need to approach performance from a different mindset than athletes without diabetes. They must be ready at any time to make corrections, i.e. use insulin. Phil continues, "I do not leave the house ever, ever without at least 100 grams of carbs and money to buy more. You just never know what might happen out there even on a 2-hour easy ride."

....

This chapter is not meant to give medical advice, replace your doctor, or be construed as health advice. Before you make ANY change, you should consult your physician.

....

This chapter attempts to provide all people with type 1 and type 2 diabetes, who are also athletes, some tips on how to use a CGM for training and competitions, and to improve their performance. If you have type 1 or type 2 diabetes and you've read this much of the book, I can imagine that you've already picked up some nuggets in the previous chapters. If you're a person without diabetes, this will be an interesting chapter for you to read and learn what people with type 1 and 2 diabetes must do to compete at a high level. You'll also realize that any type 1 diabetic competing at a high level is a serious badass. You'll also learn in this chapter what causes type 2 diabetes, how you can prevent it, and, if you have it or are prediabetic, how you can reverse it.

Type 1 diabetes, or early onset diabetes, is a condition that generally occurs in early childhood, and results from a very specific immune-mediated destruction of the pancreatic islet beta cells, and, therefore, insulin is no longer produced by the body. By definition: "Type 1 diabetes mellitus (T1D) is an autoimmune disease that leads to the destruction of insulin-producing pancreatic beta cells. Individuals with T1D require life-long insulin replacement with multiple daily insulin injections, insulin pump therapy, or the use of an automated insulin delivery system. Without insulin, diabetic ketoacidosis (DKA) develops and is life-threatening. In addition to insulin therapy, glucose monitoring with (preferably) a continuous glucose monitor (CGM) and a blood glucose monitor if CGM is unavailable is recommended."[66]

Someone with type 1 diabetes will need to inject insulin on a daily (sometimes hourly) basis to optimize glucose control. Without insulin, a person with type 1 diabetes will build up ketones to a high level, and this can become a life-threatening condition, leading to a coma or death. Ketones, as we've mentioned before, can be created by the liver out of fat in an absence of glucose, and are used by the muscles and other tissues for energy, but only if insulin is present. Since people with type 1 diabetes don't produce insulin, they're at the risk of developing ketoacidosis.

For others, it's hard to imagine how difficult it is to control your glucose levels and insulin levels with type 1 diabetes, and it's completely mind-boggling to see people with type 1 diabetes competing at professional level sports. It takes extreme control of your diet and your glucose intake, and an understanding of when to inject insulin and how much, just to be able to train effectively.

Dr. Michael Riddell PhD, professor at York University in Hamilton, Canada, is considered one of the top researchers in the field of exercise physiology/sports and type 1 diabetes. Dr. Riddell had this to say about the difficulty of living with type 1: "I have had type 1 for over 40 years now, I have published over 200 peer-reviewed journal articles, written 30 book chapters, researched type 1 diabetes for the last 25 years and I still inject the wrong amount of insulin 40% of the time as a person with type 1 diabetes. It is incredibly difficult to regulate our glucose levels in life, much less when we exercise. As a longtime cyclist and having worked with the professional cycling team, Team Novo Nordisk (formerly Team Type 1), we have found that every rider reacts a bit differently."[67]

Phil Southerland states some riders will have a completely opposite reaction than others, even before the start of a race.[68] Some riders will want to start the race with a glucose level of 200 milligrams per deciliter (mg/dL), as they know that when the race starts, their glucose will come down. Others will want to start at a glucose level of 90 mg/dL, and then feed as soon as the race starts to keep their levels stable. It's highly individual, and it also depends on the race pace, dynamics, and type.

Phil Bartels, a type 1 athlete coach for another team of athletes with type 1, a former professional for Team Type 1, and winning team member in the 2006 Race Across America in a team comprised of type 1 athletes, said, "Since we were each cycling all-out for 20–30 minutes at a time and then the next rider would 'tag in,' we had to time our glucose perfectly. We found that most of us all felt very strong with a glucose level between 140–180 mg/dL and it was better if we titrated insulin and food in order to keep us in that level. It was not easy."[69]

HYPOGLYCEMIA: HOW TO PREVENT IT FOR TYPE 1 DIABETIC ATHLETES

For athletes with type 1 diabetes, using a CGM is not just essential, but mandatory, to optimize their health and performance. CGMs were originally developed specifically for type 1 diabetics, so that they could connect with an insulin pump and work together to inject the correct amount of insulin for the glucose level. It's not foolproof, as any athlete with type 1 diabetes with this system will tell you, but it certainly has made life much easier and better. The insulin pumps now have a "sport" mode that suspends insulin doses when glucose levels drop below 100 mg/dL. The best way to prevent hypoglycemia is, firstly, to know when it can occur and, secondly, to anticipate it and take the appropriate action. Hypoglycemia can occur when:

- too much insulin is injected,
- skipping meals,
- not eating enough food that contains glucose,
- exercising more than normal, and/or
- exercising more intensely than normal.

People with type 1 diabetes are more at risk of hypoglycemia, as it's easy to inject too much insulin while exercising, causing a reactive hypoglycemic crash. At rest, it's much easier to predict the needed amount of insulin when glucose is at 150 mg/dL, as the muscles aren't requiring glucose to move and for energy. This allows the user to inject with a high degree of certainty the correct amount of insulin needed to lower glucose levels to a more realistic level, like 100–120 mg/dL, for stable energy. When exercising, glucose will be used in the muscles, and depending on the intensity of the effort, a faster reduction or slower reduction of glucose in the bloodstream will occur. At 200 mg/dL, and with immediately intense exercise, this level might naturally reduce to 100–120 mg/dL without requiring any insulin. If an athlete injects insulin right before an intense event, let's say a 5 k cross-country running event, they'll likely have a hypoglycemic crash shortly after the event starts, as the insulin has pulled the glucose out of the bloodstream instead of allowing it to be circulated and used by the muscles, which would naturally pull the glucose out of the bloodstream.

An important point to remember is that during exercise, insulin is about four times more effective than at rest, and the speed of action is also much faster. So, if one unit of insulin will give you a 50 mg/dL drop in glucose at rest, it will give you a 200 mg/dL drop at exercise. So it's very important to take care with your insulin units while exercising and to understand exactly what your glucose level is from your CGM. Caution: This is very individual, and it depends on the intensity of exercise too, so be cautious with the use of insulin during exercise. Some athletes will even wear two CGMs so they can ensure their glucose levels are as accurate as possible. Since training is critical for improvement, and glucose needs to be more tightly regulated, this could be a helpful tip for type 1 athletes.

Preventing hyperinsulinemia (too much insulin) during longer exercise can also be done by feeding more carbohydrates to "soak up" some of that extra insulin, and this is likely the most effective way to reduce insulin levels during exercise. Obviously, giving yourself less insulin in the first place is better, and reducing your injection by 50 to 80% of your normal amount 90 minutes before exercise is a good start.[70]

Is There a Difference Between the Type of Athlete and Prevention of Hypoglycemia?

Athletes that do high-intensity exercising, such as sprinting, high-intensity interval training, and even intense resistance exercise (like during a session of hard and quick exercises in CrossFit) and have type 1 may develop hyperglycemia (high blood glucose) more easily than lower intensity exercisers. During these types of exercises, which are shorter in duration, the hormonal response is similar to athletes without diabetes. See Figure 7.0. The body will elevate catecholamines, which are neurotransmitters that can cause the body to promote glucose release from the liver (gluconeogenesis) and consequently raise circulating glucose levels. Since there will be low levels of insulin in people with type 1 diabetes, then mild hyperglycemia will occur during these intense bouts.[71] Observing your CGM data during exercise is key here, so you can see exactly your glucose levels at the end of the workout. It's not suggested to inject insulin during this kind of workout, in general, unless you started with a high glucose level to begin with and then be very conservative in how much you inject.

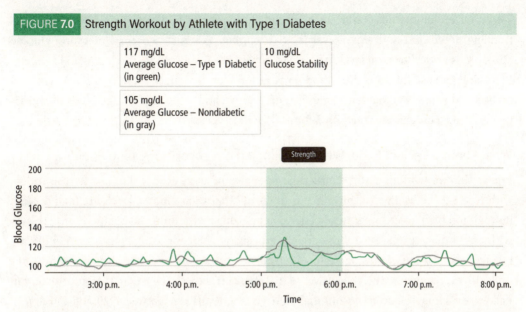

Here is an example of a strength workout done by an athlete with type 1 diabetes, showing a very similar glucose response to an athlete without diabetes.

However, a study done on post-exercise recovery with type 1 athletes stated, "the priority after finishing a bout of exercise should be to first get the blood glucose concentration of the individual stable and within the target range (73–180 mg/dL). This might be done by taking an insulin correction if required and then adding additional bolus insulin to cover the carbohydrate and protein intake consumed in early recovery to stimulate glycogen resynthesis and muscle protein synthesis. As always, it is important to reemphasize that, although the rate of glycogen resynthesis is important, the athlete with type 1 diabetes needs to balance this with the risk of hyperglycaemia and hypoglycaemia."[72] This is also critical to enhance the uptake of the glucose into your muscles for storage as glycogen, and to improve your recovery, so ensure you're getting enough insulin to cover your post-workout recovery shake and meal. At the same time, it's common for athletes with type 1 diabetes to develop hypoglycemia within 6–15 hours post-exercise (to be fair, it also happens in people without diabetes!) and this is thought to be because of the increased action of the glucose transporter type 4 (GLUT-4) transporters to the muscle cells after exercise is completed.[73] This means that if you finish a workout in the evening, it's super important to watch your CGM before you go to sleep, as you could get low during sleep, which is just a bad period, but isn't great if you're training consecutive days.

For athletes that are training and competing in endurance sports, the problem is that prolonged exercise will continue to use more and more glucose as the exercise continues.

Therefore, endurance athletes need to carefully watch their CGM, noticing when the arrow is trending downward and when levels start dropping. When this occurs, ingesting glucose (20–60 g) is critical to raise levels back up to between 140 and 180 mg/dL, and stabilize them. Managing glucose intake is even more critical for exercise longer than two hours, as many cyclists and runners compete in long-distance events, and the need for high levels of consistent and constant glucose is required for peak performance.

What About a Lack of Food, Whether Skipping a Meal or Not Eating Enough?

Preparation for working out is a critical component for every athlete, not just for the athlete with type 1 diabetes. Every athlete needs to ensure that their glucose levels are high enough (but not too high) to ensure a steady energy supply during training and competition. Athletes with type 1 diabetes have it more difficult, especially when consecutive days of training are involved, as their muscle glycogen stores replenish more slowly, and their liver glycogen stores replenish even more slowly. The answer to this question above is: Don't do it! As an athlete, you need to eat enough food to ensure that your glucose levels stay between 120 and 180 mg/dL before exercise, so that you'll have a good session. You should even consider setting an alert in your CGM app at 100 mg/dL for the hour before your workout, to ensure your glucose doesn't drop below this level. This means that you'll also need to reduce your insulin dose by 25–75%, especially if you're eating and going to train directly afterward.[74]

Dr. Michael Riddell, et.al., wrote a great paper called "Exercise Management in Type 1 Diabetes: A Consensus Statement," and I highly encourage you to read this if you're a type 1 diabetic.

Table 7.0 should help you to better decide whether you need insulin or food for exercise.[75]

WHAT ABOUT HYPERGLYCEMIA?

High blood glucose is a constant daily battle for people with type 1 diabetes, and this is where you need to be vigilant for the trends. Your CGM not only will help you train and compete at the highest level, but you'll be able to keep your energy more stable throughout the day and night, reducing high blood glucose.

The signs and symptoms of hyperglycemia include the following:[76]

- high blood glucose, which could be considered over 150 mg/dL while at rest
- high levels of glucose in the urine
- frequent urination
- increased thirst

Using your CGM, you'll have constant data to analyze and understand as you go throughout your day and training. If your blood glucose is above 240 mg/dL, you should check your urine for ketones. ***If you have ketones, do not exercise. You need insulin to reduce the glucose and ketones in your blood.*** Exercising when ketones are present may make your blood glucose level *and* ketones go even higher, and could cause ketoacidosis, which is life-threatening.

As an athlete, you can reduce high glucose by exercising. This is one of the simplest ways to reduce your glucose (besides giving insulin) and you simply need to get moving. As long as you don't have ketones, then you need to get out and go workout. Watching your CGM will also help you to reduce your glucose levels to the right amount, and thinking about the trending arrows is critical. Thinking about where you'll be in 30 minutes, rather than focusing on the current moment, is one of the best ways to manage your glucose as an athlete. For example, Phil Bartels stated, "If I had pizza before a training ride, I would not give myself the amount of insulin that my body needed at the moment, but instead I would be thinking about how much insulin my body would need to cover the carbs from the pizza during the activity. The analogy that I think of and makes great sense to me is: As a type 1 diabetic, I am driving a manual transmission car. I have to physically push in the clutch and shift the gears in order to make the car move and I need to match the right gear with the right speed. The automatic transmission car is an easier system to drive, but you don't have the ability to anticipate accelerations and decelerations like you can when driving a manual. There is a reason race car drivers use manual transmissions: they need to keep their rpms in a narrow range for maximal power, grip, and cornering ability. The good news is CGM gives you the information that your system requires to race to your top potential. For a training ride or race that comes right after a large pre-race meal like pizza, then the amount of insulin I would give would be less, and perhaps my glucose would have started to rise into "high" territory leading into the workout or race. Once the race starts, the insulin in the system will be in balance with the increased energy needs and increased sensitivity. Glucose will begin to balance out with no crash or need for additional corrections."[77]

With type 1 diabetes, you've control over when and how much insulin is delivered and, just like in a car, you need to keep the revs per minute in the right zone for optimal performance. If you do this correctly, then you might just have an advantage over non-diabetics, and you can make your body run more smoothly.

Exercising More Often than Normal and Longer than Normal

When you're used to a certain level of training, you get into a routine nutritionally, sleep-wise, and work-wise, and all of this routine helps glucose management. However, increasing your training or competition will create an additional energy requirement that won't be met with current food intake levels. This extra training demands additional glucose to create the energy you need. How will you meet these demands, and what does that mean in both the short term (1–3 days) and the longer term (4–10 days)? The first thing you need to do is to ensure that you match your carbohydrate intake to the longer workouts. If you've found that ingesting 30–60 g of carbs every hour keeps you roughly between 120 and 180 mg/dL during exercise, then ensure that you've enough carbs with you to continue that for the length of your workout, whether that's two, six, or more hours. You'll need a combination of foods and drinks to get you through those longer workouts, and you must find what works for you. Along the way, keep in mind that your injectable insulin is more powerful and faster acting than normal, so you'll continue to reduce your insulin units during the longer workouts and competitions. As you go longer and longer, the risk of developing hypoglycemia becomes more and more of an issue, so it's highly likely that you'll need to increase your carbohydrate intake, especially past five hours.

After your workouts, it's even more critical to refuel adequately. Dr. Asker Jeukendrup wrote in a recent study, "The initial rapid phase of glycogen resynthesis in the muscle appears to be because of contraction-induced GLUT4 translocation to the cell membrane and augmented glycogen synthase activity. The rate of resynthesis during this initial phase can rapidly decline in the absence of exogenous carbohydrate."[78] Here, you'll need to be careful with your insulin. You should watch your glucose, anticipate how high it will rise, and then inject enough insulin for continued uptake into the muscles to replenish the glycogen stores. While it's impractical to feed in the middle of the night, as a precaution (especially for those athletes training long periods for multiple days in a row), you should have some handy glucose tabs, gels, or bars near the bed in case you need more in the middle of the night. Doing your best to keep your glucose over 75 mg/dL while sleeping is a great goal, and one you should strive for. A study of athletes with type 1 diabetes, showed "that increasing the time in target glycemic range is a key component of getting a good night's sleep."[79] For 1–3 days of longer-than-normal training, it will be apparent that on the second and third days your base glucose level will be lower than normal, and it will require more and more ingested glucose to get your levels over 140 mg/dL. In fact, you might have to start out the workout with a high sugar energy drink, just to get the levels where you need them for a high-quality training session or competition.

Exercising More Intensely than Normal or High-Intensity Exercise

When preparing to exercise at a high-intensity level, it's important to understand the trend arrows before you begin. Phil Bartels, a former pro cyclist and type 1 diabetic on the Team Type 1 pro cycling team, put it so perfectly: "One of the most powerful features of a CGM device is the trend arrows. These tell you how quickly your blood sugar levels are climbing or falling, allowing you to predict where you will be in the future. As an athlete heading into a training session or event, this is key. Take a minute to learn what your trend arrows are telling you. How quickly are you rising or falling?"[80]

One little anecdote on this: before we had access to CGM, I remember driving to races with a van full of type 1 diabetic athletes—Phil, Joe, Bob, and myself. We would be testing our blood sugar with the traditional finger-stick method every 5 minutes leading into a race, to get a good understanding of the trend. I remember the van being littered with used test strips; it was pretty disgusting.

I also remember talking with type 1 diabetics who would complain that they felt there was no consistency in their diabetes. They would tell me stories of how they would do one thing one day and the same thing the next, with totally different results. A big reason for this feeling of unpredictability is due to the snapshot view and making a decision based on that number. To explain this more: if you are starting a bike ride and you see a BG reading of 95, the result is going to be drastically different if you are 95 heading to 300, or 95 crashing to 40. The 95 number is useless without understanding the direction. I am convinced that once you understand stress and trend arrows, diabetes becomes incredibly predictable.

Understanding how the trend is moving is absolutely critical before you knowingly begin intense exercise. This will direct how you're going to treat yourself, whether you might give a little insulin (reminder: your insulin is four times more effective during exercise, so give 75% less) or take in carbohydrates. One common mistake newer athletes can make, especially around intensity, is to inject insulin before an intense event (think: the start of a 10 k running race). It's highly likely that upon starting an intense exercise, if your glucose level is high and trending downward (over 200), it will come down even faster as the exercise starts, and as you use that glucose. You might consider injecting insulin to reduce the glucose level before you start, but that would be a mistake, as you're very likely to cause a hypoglycemic crash during your hard workout/event. If on the other hand, you're reading 120 mg/dL right before your run, and the arrow is trending flat or down, you should ingest some carbohydrates to bring up your glucose levels. If you're at 120 mg/dL and the arrow is trending up, since you just ate some carbohydrates, then that's good, as the glucose coming in will be used immediately. It's important to have some additional fast-digesting carbs to add more glucose if you see the trend arrow beginning to flatten or come down.

One critical piece of advice you should consider: try this in training first, before competition! It's difficult to simulate the adrenalin and excitement effect on your glucose levels in training, so make sure to factor that in. Competition is stress, and you need to become an expert in stress and how it impacts your blood sugar. "When stressed, the body prepares itself by ensuring that enough sugar or energy is readily available. Insulin levels fall, glucagon and epinephrine (adrenaline) levels rise, and more glucose is released from the liver. At the same time, growth hormone and cortisol levels rise, which causes body tissues (muscle and fat) to be less sensitive to insulin. As a result, more glucose is available in the bloodstream."[81] Depending on your personality and how excited you become before a race, your glucose could go up rapidly as you get closer to your event, without even exercising. If you don't get too excited about competing and are as cool as a cucumber before your event, then your glucose could remain stable, with a trend arrow that is flat, and then your decision depends on what your glucose is. If it's a little low, less than 120 mg/dL, then ingest some glucose, but if it's higher than 200 mg/dL, you're probably fine to start. Observe closely and be ready to ingest glucose if needed. Phil Bartels continued, "My CGM is a great window into your fight-or-flight system. As a T1D athlete, I learned to predict my blood sugar response based on how much adrenaline I was feeling or what other stressful life events I was experiencing."[82]

WHAT'S THE MOST IMPORTANT THING YOU CAN DO USING YOUR CGM AS A TYPE 1 DIABETIC?

Be prepared! You should always have easy and quick access to simple and complex sugars while training and competing. Be ready to eat more foods as you work out. This can be a combination of high-carb drinks and easy-to-digest bars and gels. Your goal should be to finish every training session or competition with "left over" fuel—food that you did *not* eat. This means that you had enough.

Secondly, take action! As soon as you start to see your glucose dropping below 120 mg/dL, then taking more glucose is critical to arrest this drop. This also means anticipating where you'll be in 30 minutes. Even though you see your current glucose dropping, did you just eat, and your CGM hasn't had time to update? Or, did you have a big pizza for lunch right before your gym session, and in 30 minutes your blood glucose will be through the roof, but you'll be working out then so don't give yourself too much insulin now?

There are quite a few scientific peer-reviewed published papers now, which give guidelines for competitive athletes to prevent hypoglycemia. Dr. Michael Riddell has published some guidelines for people with type 1 diabetes that are good to use. They are in Table 7.0.

WHAT ABOUT WEIGHT GAIN? CAN YOU PREVENT THIS AND WOULD A CGM HELP YOU?

This is one of the most challenging parts of being an athlete with type 1 diabetes. You need glucose to train, so you eat plenty of great carbohydrates, and then make sure you use the correct amount of insulin to keep yourself in your optimal glucose ranges. However, out on the

CHAPTER 7: Diabetes and Athletic Performance: Using a CGM

TABLE **7.0** How to Adjust Insulin and Food Intake for Exercise for People with Type 1 Diabetes		
	Aerobic exercise >30 minutes where glucose tends to drop	Anaerobic or mixed exercise lasting <30 minutes where glucose tends to rise
BEFORE EXERCISE	• Lower meal (bolus) insulin by ~50% at the meal before the activity if the exercise occurs within 120 minutes of a meal • Set a lower basal insulin rate (or a higher temp target) if using an insulin pump • If on multiple dose injection (MDI), lower total basal insulin by 20% on active days • Aim for a starting glucose of around 120–180 mg/dL • If glucose is on the lower end of target range, do some resistance exercise as a warmup	• Take usual meal (bolus) insulin at the meal before the activity if the activity occurs within 120 minutes of a meal • Maintain usual basal insulin if on an insulin pump • Aim for a starting glucose of around 90–120 mg/dL • If pre-activity is elevated, do a mild aerobic warmup (light jogging, walking, etc.)
DURING EXERCISE	• Try to maintain glucose between 120 and 180 mg/dL and consume carbohydrates as needed to maintain glucose in target range (up to 60 g per hour of exercise)	• Carbohydrates may not be needed unless glucose falls below 90 mg/dL
AFTER EXERCISE	• Take up to 50% less bolus insulin for the first meal after prolonged exercise • Monitor glucose carefully and watch for post-exercise hypoglycemia • Consider a small low-glycemic index snack (~15–20 g of carbohydrate) with some protein (~10 g protein) before bedtime, with little to no bolus insulin	• Correct any high glucose with a small amount of insulin (e.g. 50% of the usual correction dose) and an aerobic cooldown • Monitor glucose carefully and watch for post-exercise hypoglycemia • Consider a bedtime snack of low-glycemic index carbohydrate with protein with less insulin than usual • Consider a small low-glycemic index snack (~15–20 g of carbohydrate) with some protein (~10 g protein) before bedtime, with little to no bolus insulin

ride you realize you gave a little too much insulin, so now you eat more food, which raises the glucose again so you can finish your workout. After your workout, your glucose levels might drop, so you'll need to refuel (and consequently use more insulin). This might continue for a while, culminating in having to eat a meal before bed, and also giving insulin before going to sleep. Insulin promotes fat storage, so this will contribute to increased fat in the type 1 athlete. This is a really, really tough balance, as you need the right amount of glucose for energy and health, but at the same time you don't want to overdo it and gain fat.

A CGM can make a difference here in choosing the right kinds of foods post-workout to minimize your blood glucose spikes, which in turn reduces the need for insulin. The answer to this is truly in your food choices and knowing which foods will give you a large increase in glucose, which stabilize you, and which don't have impact much at all.

A great book that will help you on this path is *Mastering Diabetes* by Cyrus Khambatta and Robby Barbaro.[83] I highly recommend this book to help you keep your glucose levels in the right zone, and keep off the extra body fat.

TYPE 2 DIABETES AND THE ATHLETE

Type 2 diabetes is a very different "beast" than type 1 and is characterized by insulin resistance created by poor nutritional choices, eating more than is needed, and a lack of movement. Type 2 begins as an adult, in most cases, and when your body still produces insulin, but your cells can't use it any longer at the same levels and need more and more insulin to get the glucose out of the bloodstream and into those cells. The pancreas will produce more insulin to reduce the glucose, and eventually the beta cells within the pancreas will be used up and no longer produce insulin. In this case, the type 2 diabetic will need to inject insulin. There are many measures by which one might be considered a type 2 diabetic. The hemoglobin A1C (HbA1c) test is known as the standard to determine if you're prediabetic or diabetic. The HbA1c test looks at the average glycated blood cells over a three-month period. The HbA1c test measures how much glucose is attached to your hemoglobin blood cells. Everyone has some level of coating of glucose on their hemoglobin cells, but the more you have, the more insulin resistant you are as well. A normal HbA1c is below 5.7%, prediabetes is between 5.7% and 6.4%, and above 6.4% is considered type 2 diabetes.[84] By using your CGM, you can tell where you are on the spectrum, as an average daily glucose above 126 mg/dL is also considered type 2 diabetes. Somewhere between 110–125 mg/dL is considered prediabetes.

There are many important things to consider when you're using both of these measures to determine if you've a problem or not, especially if you're an athlete. First off, there are some people that have smaller than normal living red blood cells, which is called beta thalassemia. It's possible that some endurance athletes have this condition. If you've this condition, then your HbA1c will be higher than normal, and this test will not be valid for you. HbA1C is just an *estimate* (or *predictor*) of prevailing glucose levels, and the exact relationship between the two depends on various factors (such as red blood cell lifespan) such that it shouldn't be overinterpreted. Iron deficiency anemia can increase the life of red blood cells, and this is another example of things that can increase HbA1C.

Secondly, with your CGM, you can just look at the average glucose over 24 hours and then as an average over the last 30 days and "back" into your true HbA1c. There is a great calculator for this on the American Diabetes Association website.[85] For example, let's say that your average daily glucose over the last 30 days is 102 mg/dL. Using the calculator, your HbA1c would be 5.2%—well below the prediabetes level of 5.7%. Consider that measuring HbA1c alone might not be the most accurate solution.[86] It's important to also take into consideration that as an athlete, you're going to have plenty of time with your glucose higher than the normal sedentary person. Some athletes might exercise for four to six hours per session and that will require a much higher level of glucose to maintain energy levels. The sheer amount of time you spend at a higher level will obviously impact your daily average glucose level. The Levels app allows you to opt out of including your average blood glucose during your workouts as part of the daily average glucose, to give you a more accurate daily average glucose level. So, keep this in mind when you're looking at your daily average glucose level.

I also like to look at the nightly average glucose levels, and believe this is a good measure of where you are on the scale of HbA1c. What your average is overnight is an important indicator of how sensitive you are to insulin, and how smartly you ate the previous night. Eating too late will raise your glucose, and you might end up going to sleep with a glucose level at 140 mg/dL when you don't need that much glucose. In this case, the body most likely stores that additional glucose as fat. Eating earlier and before 8:00 p.m. is a great thing for many reasons. When you wake up and see that your average overnight was less than 100 mg/dL, then you know you're highly sensitive to insulin. On the opposite side, if you underfed, then you know it immediately when you wake up and your nightly average glucose was 75 mg/dL!

Lastly, this is a very new study of glucose levels for athletes. It's quite possible that athletes can have a much higher average glucose level without any deleterious effects, because of their high levels of metabolic fitness and health. Dr. Kristina Skroce, who has spent the last eight years working with both type 1 professional athletes and pro athletes without diabetes, had this to say, "What I genuinely believe is that PRO athletes are a separate group that doesn't fit in the 'normal' school textbooks. We're literally redefining our understanding of human physiology. I believe that elite performance requires elite glucose control. Prior to the continuous glucose visibility in CGM technology, numbers and patterns like this were seemingly impossible, designated as unhealthy. We're now saying that the current knowledge of glucose regulation in the interstitial fluid during high-intensity exercise *needs* to be challenged."[87]

What Are the Causes of Type 2 Diabetes? (It Might Be Different than You Think)

There are three main causes of type 2 diabetes. The first one is easy: eating too much. Taking in more calories than you burn will result in an overabundance of calories, and that results in

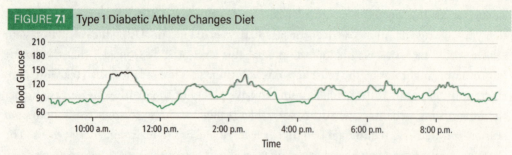

This type 1 diabetic athlete changed his diet dramatically after beginning to use a CGM. He went from being a junk food addict and having to constantly battle with his insulin and glucose levels to a very stable type 1, and much stronger athlete, by changing his diet to a more whole-food, plant-based diet. The dramatic difference took about six months of commitment, but it certainly worked. He has lost 30 lbs and kept off that extra weight, and kept his glucose levels stable, as evidenced in Figure 7.2.

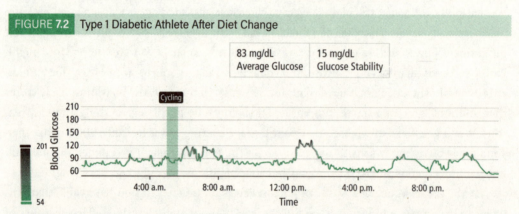

After beginning a whole-food, plant-based diet, this type 1 diabetic athlete's glucose levels are lower, more stable, and have reduced spikes.

a storage of fat. Protein and carbohydrates can be stored as fat, so it doesn't really matter what the quality of the food is that you take in, it's more about eating more than you need. Overfeeding yourself results in the storage of fat in the cells of the muscles (visceral), under the skin (subcutaneous) and the organs (visceral). Fatty liver disease, which was almost never heard of in the past, is now becoming a more and more common diagnosis. Reduce your food intake and go into a deficit where you're eating less than you expend and you'll begin to reverse type 2.

The second cause is eating too many high-glycemic foods. Notice I didn't write, "eating too many carbohydrates." We need carbs! As athletes, we eat many high-glycemic foods and drink many drinks that contain simple sugars. Simple sugars, like the kind that are in sports gels, give a great and quick boost in blood sugar when needed, but if you drink sugary sodas all day, then eat cookies, cakes and chocolate bars, you'll constantly create blood sugar spikes that will be going over 180 mg/dL throughout your day. Many staple foods are high glycemic too. It's important to *minimize* the intake of these foods, like: white rice, white and whole wheat bread, potatoes and fries, sugary breakfast cereals, potato and tortilla chips, and of course just about any food that has a lot of "added" sugar on the label. I'll give you some key strategies to employ so that you can reduce the impact of these foods on your blood sugar in Chapter 8. Eating these foods, of course, don't just cause type 2 diabetes, but it's their cumulative effect over time that will cause insulin resistance.

The third cause of type 2 diabetes is ingestion of fat. The intake of seed oils and saturated fat is a major contributor to insulin resistance. Canola oil, sunflower oil, soybean oil, etc., along with saturated fats from animal proteins (and from plant ones like avocados, just to a lesser extent) are not good for your metabolism. These fats fill up your cells, liver, organs, and muscles, and because they're full, there is no room for glucose. Obviously, this is an oversimplification of the biochemistry that happens, but we'll go further into the causes of type 2 diabetes in the next chapter.

CGMs and the Type 2 Athlete

In general, it's unlikely that many athletes at an elite level will have type 2 diabetes. As they exercise so much, it's impossible to become insulin resistant (as they're constantly burning the ingested glucose and emptying their glycogen stores regularly). However, athletes that take up a new sport as an adult might come to that sport with type 2 diabetes. If you have type 2, then how can you use your CGM to help improve your athletic performance?

The first thing that you'll notice is that your glucose zones are much higher than normal, and as a type 2 diabetic, this is expected. What this means, though, is that in training and competition, you most likely will need to maintain a higher level of glucose to perform at your optimum. Secondly, you'll notice that you're more susceptible to drops in glucose and that when you go below 120 mg/dL, you'll feel like you're getting hypoglycemic or "bonking." Again, the solution to this is to keep your glucose levels higher during exercise, vigilantly watch them, and then be ready to eat or drink foods. Third, you should consider eating and drinking more slower digesting carbs to prevent from additional spikes. This is a good thing for anyone to do, but as a type 2 diabetic, you've lower glucose tolerance, meaning your glucose will spike higher and stay higher for longer (insulin resistance). So it makes great sense to ingest slower acting and complex carbs, like a brown rice ball, a banana, or a natural sports bar with no added sugars or very low sugar (be careful about too many additives to make it "high" protein). I also recommend a slower acting carb like the starch that is in the

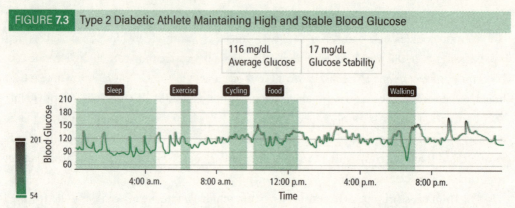

A type 2 diabetic that uses a slow-acting or complex carb to minimize glucose spikes. This athlete ingested a UCAN® sports bar and sipped on a UCAN® energy drink mix to keep his glucose levels high and stable.

UCAN® products. These are great for prediabetics and diabetics as they help to maintain more stable blood glucose values. See Figure 7.3.

There are other things that will play a large role in training and competing if you're a type 2 diabetic. These are: medications, the impact of exercise on your numbers, your weight, and your diet.

Medications like Metformin will have a big impact on your training and competition. Metformin reduces the glucose in your bloodstream, which is a good thing overall, but not great when you need that glucose to perform at your best. You might find once you start working with a CGM, that while Metformin can help you reduce the spikes and overall glucose numbers, it might be too much that you can't perform at your very best, just from a lack of available glucose. If you're taking Metformin and another drug, like Rebelsis, then you really might have a problem in increasing your glucose to a level that will give you optimal performance. One athlete that came to a cycling camp that I conducted had never used a CGM before, and had type 2. I put a CGM on him for the camp. He struggled that first day to keep his energy levels high and rode under his potential for certain. When we analyzed his CGM data after the first day, we found that his basal level was 75 mg/dL! When he had a high-glycemic sports bar, gel, or drink, it went up to 85 mg/dL—still too low. After consulting his doctor, he stopped taking the Rebelsis but stayed on the Metformin, and by the end of the week, he was able to bring his glucose up to 120–150 mg/dL, which is more of a normal range for training and competing, especially for an intense multi-day cycling camp. If you're struggling with low energy and find that once you start using a CGM as a type 2, you may have "over-corrected" your glucose levels and should speak with your doctor about possibly adjusting your dosage.

A note on glucagon-like peptide 1 (GLP-1) drugs, like Ozempic: these make it very, very difficult to train or workout at much more than an endurance pace. The side effects alone make it challenging to feel strong enough to much more than exist, but the lack of desire to eat and, therefore, the low energy levels (low glucose as well), make it nearly impossible to workout. While these drugs might be good for some people (I remain skeptical), they certainly are not good for the athlete.

Once you begin exercising, you'll find that your basal (base) glucose numbers will begin dropping, and that's a good thing. You are reversing your type 2! As you use your stored glycogen in your muscles and liver, along with using the stored fat in your cells, you'll make room for the circulating glucose and begin making your cells more insulin sensitive. Insulin begins to work properly again as you use that excess stored energy. If your normal daily average is 140 mg/dL, then you begin working out daily with enough intensity and time, you'll see your basal rate begin to reset. It's possible that after only a month of consistency, your new normal basal rate could be down near 100 mg/dL, showing that you're almost completely reversing your type 2. Now, if you're on a drug that reduces glucose, as mentioned above, you'll need to watch your CGM carefully, as it's possible that you can reduce or stop your medication altogether. Of course, talk with your doctor first and find out the best course of action. The exciting thing is that you're making great strides when you start to notice your basal average drop.

The next thing to go is your weight. As you exercise more and more, your body fat percentage should start to come down. Of course, this is still dependent on how many calories you ingest versus burn, but with a "revved-up" metabolism, you should start to burn more and more fat after your workouts, and start to see some significant weight loss. This will absolutely impact your basal average and the numbers you see while exercising. Be mindful of this so that you don't continue to put too many high-glycemic or fatty foods into your body during exercise or after, so that you continue to reduce the fat inside your cells as you burn it off with exercise.

Finally, if you're a type 2 diabetic and decide to undergo a diet change, like moving to a more whole food, plant-based diet, then you'll also begin to see reductions in your daily basal level, along with improvements in your insulin sensitivity. A whole food, plant-based diet is an excellent choice for anyone wanting to reverse type 2, as the elimination of ultra-processed foods, reduction in saturated fats, and lowered ingestion of added sugars will make a big difference in ridding your cells of excess fats and essentially creating space for glucose to be removed from the bloodstream. A whole food, plant-based diet is not the only way to improve your basal glucose level; a simple reduction in calories will also help reduce your glucose levels and excess body fat. However, it's critical that you reduce your oil and saturated fat intake.

Analyzing your CGM data will demonstrate a new lower basal glucose level, but it will take time, of course, so don't expect results overnight. When you observe that you've lowered glucose levels, understand that the same principles apply that we have addressed so far in this book, but now you're more glucose tolerant, so you'll see a lower-level increase in glucose, and a faster return to your basal level.

The important point in all these factors that impact your glucose levels as a type 2 is that you need to monitor your CGM to understand what is happening with your glucose, and then take appropriate action. This might mean ingesting enough glucose to sustain a higher level of glucose, or it might mean resetting your glucose zones as your insulin sensitivity has improved.

| | CHAPTER 8 |

Using Your CGM for Longevity and Vitality

YOU'VE SPENT MOST OF THIS BOOK learning about how to use a continuous glucose monitor (CGM) for the improvement of your athletic performance. If you're in your twenties, thinking about how long you'll live and your quality of life might seem like a distant concern. It's hard to even think about how you could extend and improve both your longevity and vitality. However, for those older than 50, and for whom the ageing process is kicking in, it's increasingly important to consider these things if you want to keep living life to the fullest. For both these age groups, and those in between, taking steps to increase your longevity (how long you live) and improve your vitality (your quality of life) is something that you can do every day in your daily choices. You're already doing one of the biggest things right now to help: exercising regularly. This *must* continue throughout your life. I hope you'll continue to make it a priority, no matter how busy you are now or become in the future.

The other "lever" that you can move is your nutritional lever. I would argue that this is not quite as important as the physical activity lever, but it's a close second. There are many other levers you can move, but in general, the benefits of these pale compared to exercise and diet. For certain, meditation, sleep, reducing or eliminating alcohol, increasing your social interactions, playing outside more, and even flossing your teeth, can contribute to a longer life with more energy.

This book would not be complete if I didn't give you sound strategies to use with your CGM, and information on how you can tell you're improving your longevity and vitality. A CGM, as you now know, is an incredible tool for enhancing performance, and it can, and should, be used in the rest of your life, as well as to improve all aspects of your life. First, we need to ensure you truly understand how to prevent and eliminate type 2 diabetes, as reducing the chances of becoming a type 2, and/or reversing type 2, is a guaranteed way to improve your longevity and vitality.

WHAT ARE THE CAUSES OF TYPE 2?

In the previous chapter, we outlined the three main causes of type 2 diabetes, so let's review them:

1. Overfeeding or eating more calories than you're expending
2. Eating too many high-glycemic foods
3. Ingesting too many saturated fats from animal and plant proteins and oils, including seed oils

Overeating can contribute to your body storing more fat for certain, and while the biochemistry of how that occurs is complicated, it's helpful to understand some of the basics. One concept that is important to understand when you think about storing more fat is where you store the fat. You might have met some obese people that have perfectly good glucose levels and are not prediabetic or type 2 diabetic. How can this be? Don't all obese people have diabetes? This is obviously not the case, and where fat is stored in the body is significant. Where you store is a cause of insulin resistance, and different people are predisposed to store fat in different areas of the body. When your body stores more fat in the subcutaneous fat (these people will be more pear-shaped), you're less likely to have insulin resistance. When these people overfeed themselves, they store fat as new molecules of fat, instead of just increasing the size of the existing fat cells, which is called hyperplasia. Eventually, there is a limit to this storage location, and you'll run out of preadipocytes. Preadipocytes are cells that are in "waiting," which can become fat cells (adipocytes) if existing fat cells become completely saturated. If you overfeed yourself, carbohydrates can convert into fat cells, but more so they contribute to storing ingested fat, so the fat you ingest *with* the carbohydrates is more likely to be stored. This process is called *de novo* lipogenesis. When this occurs, the existing fat cells will begin to increase in size. As fat cells increase in size, their ability to receive oxygen is reduced and some cells will die, which is not a healthy thing. These fat cells can then call for "help" and monocytes come along and clean up the dead fat cells. Monocytes can build new blood vessels to transport more oxygen to the fat cells, and even create cytokines that help to make them more insulin resistant, which stops their growth and protects them from death.[88] So, in this context, insulin resistance is a "self-preservation" mechanism for the fat cells. When that fat cell is as large as it can get, if glucose, fatty acids, and insulin come along, insulin can no longer shuttle glucose and fatty acids into the fat cells, which would make them too big to survive, so again, protecting the fat cell from death. At the same time, these fat cells can't inhibit the release of fatty acids from that fat cell (which usually only happens during fasting). Therefore, fatty acids are constantly being released into the bloodstream. The fat cell is trying to reduce the number

CHAPTER 8: Using Your CGM for Longevity and Vitality   131

of fatty acids in it to get back to a more normal size. If you have your blood tested, and your triglyceride levels are high, then this could be what is happening within your cells. While the preservation of fat cells' lives is now occurring, insulin resistance has been created in the subcutaneous fat tissue, which is bad, as subcutaneous fat tissue is one place that can remove sugar out of the bloodstream.

The second place that you can store fat is in the visceral fat, deep within the body (these people are more apple-shaped). People who store fat here are more likely to have insulin resistance. It's not that storing more visceral fat causes insulin resistance, but it means that the subcutaneous fat in these people is filled to capacity and can no longer store more fat. At this point, fat begins to store in the liver, organs, muscles, and between the organs. This is called ectopic fat or fat that is stored in places that are not really made for this purpose. The cells in the organs and muscles take up glucose after meals. They then become increasingly full of fat and can't take up more glucose (the same problem above), so insulin resistance is even greater.

Keep in mind that just because someone has increased their body fat or is obese, that does not necessarily cause insulin resistance. It's where the fat is stored. Once you overwhelm the storage of subcutaneous fat and begin storing fat in the visceral areas, that's when insulin resistance occurs. As your body fat percentage becomes higher and higher, at a certain point, you'll crossover to storing fat in the visceral areas. Where that crossover is, can be very individual. This is called the "personal fat threshold"[89] hypothesis and is put forth by many scientists, including Dr. Mario Kratz, whose work has focused on metabolic diseases.

The second cause is eating too many high-glycemic foods. Notice I didn't write, "eating too many carbohydrates." We need carbs! As athletes, we eat many high-glycemic foods and drink many drinks that contain simple sugars. Simple sugars, like the kind that are in sports gels, give a great and quick boost in blood sugar when needed, but if you drink sugary sports drinks all day, then eat cookies, cakes and chocolate bars, you'll constantly create blood sugar spikes that will go over 180 milligrams per deciliter (mg/dL). Many staple foods are high glycemic too; it's important to *minimize* the intake of these, including white rice, white and whole wheat bread, potatoes and fries, sugary breakfast cereals, potato and tortilla chips, and, of course, just about any food that has a lot of "added" sugar on the label.

Eating these foods, of course, doesn't just cause type 2 diabetes, but it's their cumulative effect over time that will cause insulin resistance. By having constantly high glucose levels, you'll quickly saturate the muscle and liver cells, as they can only turn so much glucose into glycogen. Once these are full, ingesting additional sugars will only cause that glucose to be converted into fatty acids, which are eventually synthesized into triglycerides, and then stored in the fat cells, making them larger and larger (which you just learned about). To reiterate and clarify, eating too many (an excess of) high-glycemic foods can cause insulin resistance. This takes time but is clearly one of the causes. I don't want you to get the wrong idea here either, and just cutting out all carbs is *not* the answer, especially as an athlete. You *must have* carbohydrates to train and compete intensely. It's more about cutting out, or significantly reducing, your intake of high-glycemic foods that matters, especially before and after you exercise.

The third cause of type 2 diabetes is fat. This is similar to what was just written above, but I want to call this out specifically as a third cause because it's so important, and many people don't put two and two together in understanding that the ingestion of fat plays a large role. The intake of oils (specifically seed oils) and saturated fat from animal proteins is a major contributor to insulin resistance. Canola oil, sunflower oil, soybean oil, etc., along with saturated fats from animal proteins (and also from plant ones like avocados, just to a lesser extent) are not good for your cell metabolism. They are, however, better for you than animal fats, including beef tallow. These fats fill the cells in the process of lipogenesis as these are already in "fat" form and are more readily stored in the existing cells. Imagine fats (in the form of triglycerides) and glucose that you've eaten being circulated in your bloodstream. They come to the cell wall, asking to be let in. The insulin your pancreas has secreted is the "key" that unlocks the door to the cell and allows the fat and glucose inside. Some more fat and glucose come along, and this time, the cell says, "We have enough glucose, but we can take in some more fat," so the fat shuttles inside the cell, this time filling the cell completely with glucose and fats. More fats and glucose come along and knock on the door of the cell, but this time the key (insulin) doesn't work anymore, as the cell "locks" the door and says, "We're full, come back another time." This is insulin resistance. The insulin is no longer effective in getting the glucose and/or fats into the cell, and the glucose continues to circulate in your bloodstream raising your glucose levels (which you see on your CGM), along with your triglyceride levels. At this point in the process, there is nowhere for the glucose to go, and it just continues to circulate until a) more insulin is released, which forces the door open, or b) you use the excess glucose with activity. What's the cause? It's the fat you ingested. It's the seed oils in your foods, and it's the saturated fats in your protein sources. Cut out those fats and you'll make your cells healthy again as you burn off the fats inside your cells and don't replace them with more fats.

GLUCOSE TOLERANCE

I haven't mentioned much about glucose tolerance, except for in Chapter 6 with the case study, so let's go deeper into this concept here, as it applies to improving your metabolic health. What is glucose tolerance? What is glucose intolerance?

Glucose tolerance is the ability of your body to dispose of glucose into your tissues and cells after you ingest it.[90] You might eat a high-carbohydrate meal, like pasta with red sauce or brown rice with corn and beans, causing your glucose to rise to a peak. How tall that peak is, whether it goes to 140 mg/dL or 190 mg/dL *and* how long it stays up there before returning to your basal level, determines how well you tolerate glucose. There is a standard test called the oral glucose tolerance test (OGTT), which involves ingesting 75 g of glucose (six tablespoons!) and then monitoring how well your body handles the glucose. Taking your blood glucose level before ingestion and after having fasted for 12 hours, drinking the syrupy solution, and then retesting your glucose after two hours, will give a clear indication of your ability to dispose of glucose throughout your tissues. At the two-hour point, your glucose should be below 140 mg/dL if you have a "normal" glucose regulation. If it's between 141 and 199 mg/dL, you might have prediabetes. If it's *over* 200 mg/dL at two hours, then you're considered to have diabetes.

Glucose intolerance is considered the root cause of blood sugar spikes. Well, insulin resistance is actually the root cause, of course, but it's also considered to be glucose intolerance. What does glucose intolerance look like? In Figure 8.0 we see an athlete that hasn't been diagnosed with prediabetes or diabetes but has glucose intolerance, and is clearly on the path to prediabetes. How can you tell?

Glucose peaks or spikes are physiological, and you shouldn't worry about small increases in glucose. Just because you have a rise in your glucose, doesn't mean you're diabetic or going to become diabetic. Everyone has some sort of rise in their glucose levels after a meal, and as long as this increase doesn't last for very long (greater than one hour), then really there is nothing to worry about. A very high peak of glucose could be due to fast gastric emptying, or just a small delay in the initial insulin response. See Figure 8.1 for an example of someone with good glucose tolerance.

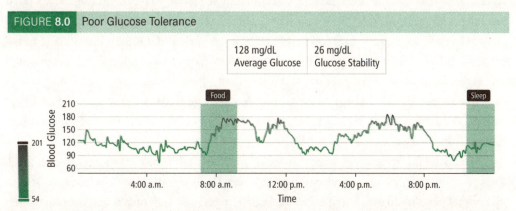

FIGURE 8.0 Poor Glucose Tolerance

Notice how when he has a glucose spike that it goes up fairly high, in most cases over 160 mg/dL, and it stays high for a while before slowly coming down. This is a sure indicator of poor glucose tolerance, and insulin resistance. Not enough insulin resistance to raise his HbA1c, but enough to be concerned about.

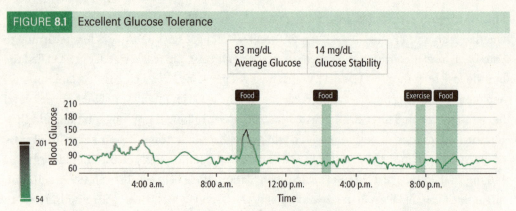

FIGURE 8.1 Excellent Glucose Tolerance

This is a great example of someone with excellent glucose tolerance. See the spike to 150 mg/dL after breakfast but the rapid return to basal rate? That's what you are striving for! Reminder: this is just an example; the response will depend on the meal type, composition, timing, and quantity, and individual insulin sensitivity.

THE SECOND MEAL EFFECT

The second meal effect is an interesting effect that occurs in your second meal of the day that contains carbohydrates. The carbs that you eat at one meal actually help to lower your glucose response from the carbs eaten in the second meal. When you have carbohydrates for breakfast, your body releases insulin to deal with that glucose and then is prepared with a small amount of insulin "at the ready" for the second meal containing carbs. This is called an "early phase insulin response," and this can also be impacted by levels of free fatty acids and the incretin hormone.[91] Not only does the early first phase of insulin response contribute to this second meal effect, but it's also thought that indigestible carbohydrates contribute too.[92] What are indigestible carbohydrates? Resistant starches are like carbohydrate-rich foods that have been allowed to cool, such as potatoes and pasta. (You'll learn more about retrogradation later in the chapter.) Other sources are parts of the soluble fibrous foods that contain gums, pectins, and mucilages, found in barley, oats, beans, and fruits. Lastly, there are indigestible carbohydrates in insoluble fiber as well, called hemicellulose, cellulose, and lignin that are in whole grains and vegetables. These insoluble fibers add bulk to your stool and help promote the feeling of fullness (satiety) from foods.

What does this mean in practical terms for you? First off, if you have a higher-carb meal, then your next higher-carb meal will have a lower glucose spike than the first one. It also means that you should not switch back and forth between low-carb meals, that contain mainly protein and fats, and higher-carb meals. This will really increase your glucose level for the second meal.

WHY IS MAINTAINING STABLE GLUCOSE IMPORTANT FOR YOUR BODY?

There are many reasons why you would like to reduce the height of your glucose spikes and the length of time your glucose is over 140 mg/dL. When you have the chance to reduce the peaks by making a better choice in foods, then you should do that. For example, if you just eat "naked" carbs (carbs without any proteins, fats or fiber) for breakfast, like a packet of oatmeal, then you might send your glucose to 180 mg/dL for an hour or more. See Figure 8.2 for an example of this. But, if you add in ground flaxseeds, hemp hearts, organic almond butter for some healthy fats, some fruits with fiber, and some unsweetened plant milk, your glucose may only rise to 120 mg/dL and stay more stable for longer. See Figure 8.3 for an example of how to mediate your glucose spike.

Keeping your glucose more stable means that there is less production of insulin by your pancreas. The beta cells that produce the insulin in your pancreas can become "exhausted" if you spend a lifetime on a glucose roller coaster, and you could end up developing type 1.5 diabetes. This is diabetes that occurs later in life and is characterized by a lowered, if not completely absent, production of insulin by the pancreas. It's something you want to avoid!

Higher glucose levels, over 140 mg/dL, are proven to do damage to the endothelial cells on the inside of the walls of your arteries.[93] Damaging these protective cells is similar to punching a hole in the inside wall of your home. If there is a hole in the wall, what do you do? You take some plaster and other materials and patch that hole. That's the role that cholesterol plays in your arteries. You can think of the low-density lipoproteins (LDLs) as the plaster (plaque) that come along patching up the weakened areas in your arteries. If you continue to stress and damage those endothelial cells with high glucose levels, more and more plaque builds up,

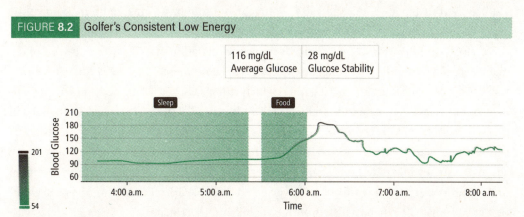

FIGURE 8.2 Golfer's Consistent Low Energy

This golfer complains about consistent low energy about an hour and a half after breakfast, which aways coincides with the 5th or 6th hole on the golf course. He eats two packets of oatmeal each morning, which are considered "naked" carbs.

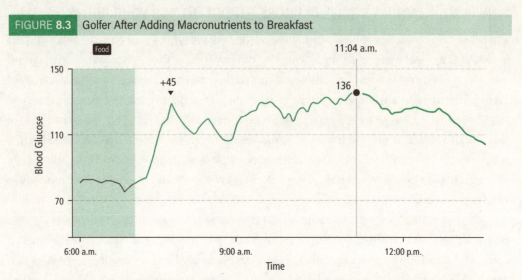

The same golfer has now added other macronutrients to his oatmeal, like ground flaxseeds, fruits, and unsweetened plant milk, to help mediate his glucose spike, and keep his glucose level more stable for his entire golf round.

eventually causing a blockage.[94] Not good! This is a very oversimplified explanation of a complicated biochemical process inside your body, but nonetheless, it's one cause of additional plaque buildup in the arteries.

Ingestion of glucose-rich foods and the circulation of more glucose in your bloodstream can create advanced glycation end products (AGEs). As you've read before and noticed in your CGM data, increasing your load of high-glycemic and glucose-rich foods cause a higher level of glucose in your bloodstream and raises your glucose numbers. This additional glucose is attached to your hemoglobin cells, which the hemoglobin A1C (HbA1c) test measures, and is called glycation. Glycation of the cells leads to the accumulation of AGEs, which are one of the main factors contributing to the ageing process.[95] What do these AGEs do to you? This glycation causes proteins to cross-link together, which stiffens tissues in our body, most concerningly our arteries and the heart muscle itself. This impaired elasticity can result in high blood pressure, peripheral artery disease, heart disease, and even cancer.[96] (Stiffness of breast tissue is associated with a higher risk of cancer.)[97] Advanced glycation end products also create chronic, systemic inflammation. There are receptors in our body for AGEs that can set off an inflammatory cascade, and researchers have named these RAGE: receptors for advanced glycation end products.[98] When AGEs set off RAGE, inflammatory genes are triggered, along with the promotion of further RAGE expression, which leads to a feedback cycle that can contribute to the development of chronic noninfectious diseases.[99] Not good! AGEs may even accumulate in our bones, joints, and muscles, and contribute to osteoporosis, arthritis, and sarcopenia, which causes the loss of muscle mass as we age.[100] The list goes on, with AGEs implicated in age-related memory loss, cataracts, Alzheimer's disease, and erectile dysfunction.[101] Suffice it to say that just this reason alone should make you want to reduce your glucose load and ensure that you have a good glucose tolerance!

As an aside, I would be remiss not to mention that AGEs are created from heat, and just body heat is enough to create them. They're also created during cooking food, specifically animal proteins. Researchers found that the highest levels of AGEs were in "high-heat-treated meat" and also in animal-derived proteins that are high in fat and protein. The lowest levels were found in vegetables, fruits, whole grains and milk.[102] What about meat? Meat can average more than 20 times more AGEs than highly processed foods, and 150 times more than fruits and veggies. Think chicken is better? Wrong. Chicken and turkey are the worst, with 20 times more AGEs than beef.[103]

How Do You Reduce AGEs?

The easiest and best way to reduce AGEs is to cut down or cut out animal-derived proteins, and lower the temperature at which you cook your foods. High-dry heating is the worst, with "oven-frying meat worse than deep-frying, which is worse than broiling, which is worse than roasting. The safest way of cooking meat are lower temperature moist methods, like boiling, poaching, stewing and steaming."[104] What about veggies and fruits? According to the most excellent book, *How Not to Die* by Dr. Michael Greger, and a study looking at the AGEs of different foods, "Even a baked apple will have more AGEs than a raw one. A raw one has 13, whereas baking an apple creates 45 AGEs. What about boiling a hot dog? A boiled hot dog has 6,736 AGEs. If you broil a hot dog on high heat, this is even worse and creates 10,143 AGEs.[105] So, a baked apple will have 150 times less AGEs than a broiled hot dog."[106] There are studies showing that the drug, Acarbose, which when taken blocks our starch and sugar digesting enzymes in the digestive tract, slows the carbohydrate absorption in our body, and even reduces AGEs by 30% over a 12-week period.[107] I know this short digression doesn't have much to do with your CGM or glucose, but it's important enough that you should know about it, for your longevity and vitality's sake!

Keto Is *not* the Answer

As I've mentioned previously in this book, "going keto" or cutting out all carbs is not the answer to improved athletic performance, and it's definitely *not* the answer to increased longevity and vitality. With what you've just read, you might think that cutting out carbs completely is the answer. It's not. While cutting out carbs completely in the short term will absolutely reduce your glucose levels, reduce your body fat, and for those that have 30 lbs or more to lose, even improve your lipids, this only will last temporarily. I will even go so far as to say that if you've *over* 50 lbs to lose, then going keto is a decent way to "jump-start" your fat loss. Keep in mind this is a *temporary fix*, and you're still filling your fat cells with fats and creating insulin resistance, you just don't know it because your glucose levels are stable because you aren't eating any carbohydrates. Once you've spent six to ten months going keto, you need to shift to become metabolically healthy and ensure that the cells in your organs, liver, and muscles are also healthy. This means reducing the proteins and fats and increasing the carbohydrates, but doing it with healthy, whole, plant-based foods. Eating plenty of fibrous and healthy vegetables will help you to continue your body fat loss, as these foods are not calorically dense but do fill the stomach, providing satiety. This is imperative if you decide to go this route in weight loss. Again, the problem with this is that your workouts will really suffer, and it will be very difficult to do any intense, higher heart-rate work that's above roughly 85% of your threshold heart rate.[108] No one is arguing that you can do lower-intensity workouts, like riding your bicycle for eight or more hours at a low intensity, without carbs, and certainly, if you're sedentary, you can live without carbs, as your liver will create glucose for usage in a process called gluconeogenesis. However, if you plan on doing any intense workout, you'll need glucose to fuel your muscles.

The Correct Answer

There are two ways that I recommend reducing your glycemic load, which will reduce your glucose spikes, help you to maintain a more stable amount of glucose in your bloodstream, and improve the metabolic health of your cells. These are: start eating lower-glycemic foods and move toward a whole food, plant-based diet.

What are low-glycemic foods and what does that mean? These are foods that have lower rates of glucose absorption based on the glycemic index (GI). All foods are ranked in the GI, which was created in the early 1980s by Dr. David Jenkins. The rates at which foods raise your blood glucose level are ranked compared to the absorption of 50 g of pure glucose. 50 g (4 tablespoons) of pure glucose is the reference value and has a GI of 100. In the GI, foods are considered "low" if they've a ranking of 55 or lower, "medium" from 56–69 and "high" if 70 and above. Low-glycemic foods are foods that have more fiber in them, both soluble and insoluble, are more slowly digested and absorbed, and, as a consequence, cause a slower rise in glucose and also a smaller rise in insulin. You wouldn't spike so quickly nor as high! There are numerous factors that influence the GI rating of foods, and these include: how refined the carbohydrate is, the composition of the nutrients within the food, the cooking method, the ripeness of the food, the structure of the starch, and the predominant sugar it contains. For example, an unripe banana will have a GI of around 30, but a ripe one will have a GI of 48. Adding some healthy fats, like ground flaxseeds and hemp hearts, to your cereal in the morning could reduce your GI from 60 to 35. The processing of foods strips away the important fiber content and raises the GI. For example, whole wheat bread that contains 12 types of seeds has a GI of 65, whereas white bread has a GI of 90. Have a look at the different GIs of foods on https://glycemic-index.net. Here are some great low-glycemic foods that athletes should eat:

- Strawberries: 41
- Dates: 42
- Oranges: 43
- Bananas: 51
- Mangos: 51
- Sweet potatoes (boiled): 63
- Pumpkins (boiled): 74
- Barley: 28
- Quinoa: 53
- Rolled oats: 55
- Couscous: 65
- Popcorn: 65
- Brown rice: 68
- Soybeans: 16
- Kidney beans: 24
- Chickpeas: 28
- Lentils: 32
- Soymilk: 34
- Skim milk: 37
- Whole milk: 39
- Ice cream: 51

Does eating low glycemic help? Absolutely! You can lower the height of your glucose spikes and their length by adding these low-glycemic foods into your diet. Here is a simple test that you can do today or any time: try eating one cup of white rice for breakfast one morning, ensuring that you ate a healthy dinner the night before and finished eating before 7:00 p.m. See what your glucose goes to and how long it takes to return to your previous level. Do the same the following morning and use one cup of brown rice. Now, what happens to your glucose levels?

What about a whole food, plant-based diet (WFPB)? This is by far the best intervention you can implement to reduce your glucose spikes, reduce

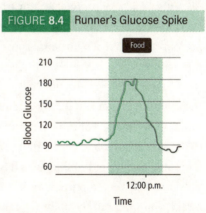

FIGURE 8.4 Runner's Glucose Spike

A glucose response from a runner that ate an almond butter, jelly, and white bread sandwich.

your risk of cancers, cardiovascular disease, stroke, and many noninfectious diseases, along with dramatically increasing your longevity and vitality. The popularity of WFPB nutrition continues to grow as more and more awareness of the benefits of this diet reaches more people. There are entire books on this subject, and the evidence is so compelling across many areas for improving longevity and vitality. One book that you should absolutely put on your reading list if you're serious about improving your longevity and vitality is *How Not to Age* by Dr. Michael Greger—it's excellent, five stars. In fact, it has been referenced many times in this book. When embarking on a WFPB, it's important that you eat "whole foods," as many people become vegetarians or vegans for health reasons, only to become "junk-food" vegetarians

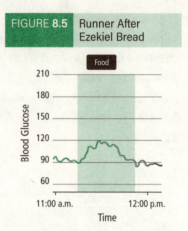

The glucose response from the same runner, but just using Ezekiel bread instead, which is a great choice for a low-glycemic bread.

or vegans. Instead of buying whole vegetables, fruits, grains, and legumes, they continue to purchase processed and ultra-processed plant foods in boxes and containers. These same people then wonder why their lipid panels haven't reduced, or their HbA1c hasn't gone down. As an athlete, you'll definitely want to ensure that you're getting enough complex carbohydrates through grains and legumes, as these will be critical to ensure your glycogen stores are full, and then replenish them after hard workouts. The most common question that vegetarians and vegans get is: "Where do you get your protein?" This isn't an issue if you eat a WFPB. All vegetables have protein, and nearly all of them are complete proteins, they just don't contain all the nine essential amino acids in similar ratios, so it's still important to combine your protein sources.[109] It's not important to combine protein sources in a single meal, although that's perfectly fine to do.[110] If you've beans, peppers, zucchini, and roasted eggplant at lunch, then have salad, corn, brown rice and tempeh at dinner, your body will be able to combine those amino acids from dinner and lunch to form the other amino acids your body needs to function optimally. For those of you that don't know where to get proteins in foods, then look to beans! Legumes like beans, split peas, chickpeas, and lentils are all power-packed with proteins and low in methionine, which is much higher in animal proteins. Methionine has been proven to be a very important amino acid for cancer growth, and by reducing your methionine intake, you snuff out the ability of cancer cells to grow.[111] The methionine content of tissues is also highly linked to maximum lifespan among mammals. The lower the methionine, the longer the longevity.[112]

CHAPTER 8: Using Your CGM for Longevity and Vitality   141

If you are worried about protein, then make sure that you have some tempeh, tofu, or unsweetened soy milk daily, and if you're exceedingly concerned, adding a plant-based protein shake is perfectly fine. Before you do that, I would suggest you log your food in an app, like Cronometer, to see how many grams of protein you're getting daily. The RDA suggested amount is 0.8 g per kg of body weight. I believe that if you're an endurance athlete, you should strive for 1.0 to 1.2; if you are a bodybuilder, 1.2 to 1.5 g per kg of body weight is plenty. Most people who believe they are on a "normal" diet get between 1.0 and 1.2 grams of protein per kg without even trying, and this includes WFPB eaters. It's just not the issue that you've been told it is.[113]

ACTIONS YOU CAN TAKE RIGHT NOW TO IMPROVE YOUR LONGEVITY AND VITALITY, REDUCE YOUR BLOOD GLUCOSE SPIKES, AND GAIN INSULIN SENSITIVITY

1. **Food stacking.** A simple yet surprising way that you can have an immediate effect on your blood glucose increases is by "stacking" your food. This is a way of eating your food in a particular order that slows down your digestion and thereby reduces your blood sugar spike.

   a. It goes like this:

      i. Always include a fresh salad with your lunch and dinner and eat this first. Use a tiny bit of olive oil and more balsamic vinegar (you'll learn about vinegar in number 7).

      ii. Eat all your vegetables next. Don't eat some veggies, and then some carbs and some proteins. Eat *all* your veggies and nothing else. Finish them off.

      iii. Now, you can eat your main protein source, whatever that happens to be. Again, eat this all at once and finish it off.

      iv. Finally, you can tackle your carbs. Eat all your carbs, they're a dessert anyhow!

If you stack your food in your belly with this method, you'll slow down your digestion, ensure a lower glucose spike, and maintain a more stable glucose for longer.

2. **Eat foods after they've undergone retrogradation.** When you cook starchy foods like potatoes, rice and pasta and eat it right away, all those carbs can easily be digested into individual glucose molecules, and then raise your blood glucose quickly. However, if you cool those starches down, in a fridge and preferably overnight, then some of that starch will be converted into resistant starch, which can't be digested. This means that the amount of glucose that enters the bloodstream will be lower. Double bonus:

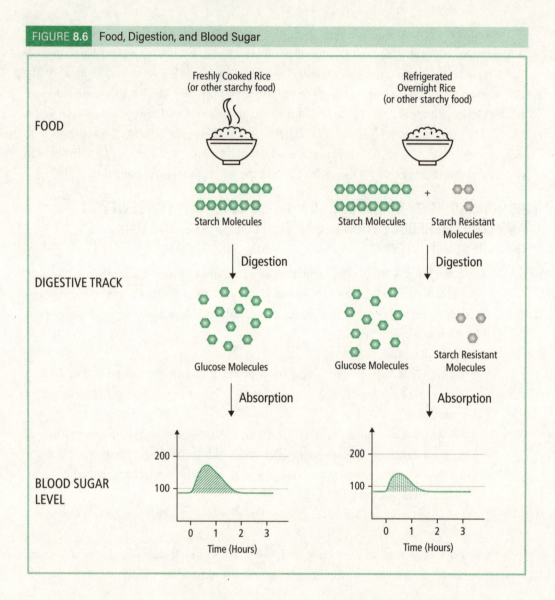

FIGURE 8.6 Food, Digestion, and Blood Sugar

once that starch has been converted into a resistant starch it can't be converted back into a digestible starch, so it's fine to reheat it and enjoy! Just remember that having some resistant starch doesn't turn your frozen french fries into a health food!

3. **Incorporate amla powder into your meals or drinks.** Amla is Indian gooseberry, and is known as one of the most antioxidant-rich foods on Earth.[114] It's not very common in Western countries but has been extensively used in India and surrounding countries

CHAPTER 8: Using Your CGM for Longevity and Vitality   143

for hundreds, if not thousands, of years. It has been the subject of hundreds of articles in medical studies examining everything from reducing cancer and cholesterol levels to improving arterial function and glucose tolerance. In Ayurvedic medicine, amla is considered "the best medicine to increase the lifespan."[115] Amla has been shown to reduce triglycerides and cholesterol,[116] reduce markers of oxidative DNA damage[117] and reduce inflammation,[118] and, most importantly from our perspective, improve the blood glucose control (tolerance) in diabetics *and* non-diabetics.[119]

4. **Eliminate seed oils, ultra-processed food and junk food from your diet.** Seed oils are oils that come from processed seeds, including canola, soybean, sunflower, sesame, cottonseed, peanut, palm kernel, corn, safflower, rice bran, and grapeseed. These are the most common seed oils used in many, many processed and ultra-processed foods today. It's nearly impossible to pick up *any* box in a grocery store that does not contain one of these oils. Not only are they in processed and ultra-processed foods, but most restaurants also use them for sauteing, deep-frying, and grilling. These polyunsaturated fatty acids (PUFAs) omega-6 fat linoleic acids are thought to play an important role in atherosclerosis formation. The ingestion of these oils after oxidation through heating and exposure to the oxygen of linoleic acid is associated with coronary artery disease.[120] While the intake of omega-6 linoleic acids from food sources like nuts, legumes, and olive oil have shown protection against developing type 2 diabetes (with energy from these sources replacing refined carbs), those from pressed and processed oils could be causal in the creation of insulin resistance.[121] Junk food and fast food contain saturated fats, PUFAs, and highly refined carbohydrates that not only lead to a rise in glucose levels, but they help to maintain high levels for longer, decreasing your glucose tolerance. The chronic consumption of seed oils, highly refined carbohydrates, and ultra-processed foods increases your glucose levels without giving your body the nutrients and fiber it needs to perform optimally.

5. **Minimize high-glycemic foods.** By now, you should know that high-glycemic foods raise your blood glucose quickly and can lead to reactive hypoglycemic crashes, putting stress on your metabolic system, not to mention sending you on a roller coaster of energy and mood swings. Absolutely, you'll need high-glycemic sports gels, bars, and drinks just before, during, and even after training and competition to enhance performance. However, these are used in a small duration of your day. In the rest of your life, ingestion of high-glycemic foods should be minimized to help increase your longevity and vitality.

6. **Start a whole food, plant-based diet.** Moving toward a more plant-based diet over time will make a difference in reducing chronic inflammation, protecting against

heart disease, protecting against certain cancers, and preventing you from becoming insulin resistant. There are so many books written on this topic and the benefits of a plant-based diet, that the evidence is incontrovertible. Hundreds, if not thousands, of peer-reviewed studies have shown the benefits of plants in your diet. A major Harvard study showed that "when plant-based proteins are consumed instead of protein from beef, poultry, fish, dairy products, or eggs, mortality is reduced."[122] If you're not plant-based now, take some steps toward becoming more and more plant-based. It takes time to learn how to cook and eat meals that are not centered around animal proteins. I have spent over two years transitioning toward a plant-based diet and can't say that I'm 100% plant-based, as I still occasionally eat seafood and venison. The changes have been profound in my average daily glucose numbers since embarking on this new way of eating. In Figure 8.7, you can see just how dramatically my average daily glucose has dropped, making me more insulin sensitive, lowering my HbA1c, ApoB (Apolipoprotein B-100), homocysteine levels, and Triglyceride to HDL (high density lipoprotein) ratios. If this inspires you, I suggest you go now to get some baseline blood testing done so that you can compare your numbers before plant-based and during. I recommend testing those markers I mentioned above as a great place to start, as these could be now considered the gold standard in testing for metabolic health. It's worth repeating and the studies prove it. "You can't out-exercise a bad diet."[123]

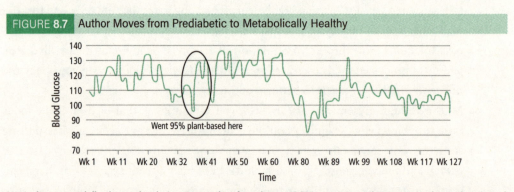

FIGURE 8.7 Author Moves from Prediabetic to Metabolically Healthy

Hunter's average daily glucose levels over 31 months of continuous CGM usage. Note that upon starting a plant-based diet at week 35, his average daily glucose levels actually went up! This is normal as he consumed more fruits and carbohydrates in general. At week 70, look at the incredible change in average daily glucose. He went from averaging 125 mg/dL per day to 105 mg/dL. This moved him from being considered clinically prediabetic to a normal, insulin-sensitive, metabolically healthy person.

7. **Have some apple cider vinegar before your meal, and squeeze lemon/lime juice in your water.** Apple cider vinegar (ACV) can increase your postprandial (meal) insulin sensitivity by 34%.[124] ACV has also been shown to reduce HbA1c levels in individuals with type 2 diabetes.[125] ACV contains acetic acid which, when consumed 5 to 30 minutes before a carbohydrate meal, can reduce your blood glucose spike and levels. There are multiple mechanisms thought to be at work here: the inhibition of the alpha-amylase action, which is secreted in the mouth and helps to slow down starch digestion; increased glucose uptake by cells and mediation by transcription factors, all which somewhat mimic the effects of the drugs acarbose and Metformin. A very well-designed study not only showed that ACV reduced postprandial high blood glucose and high

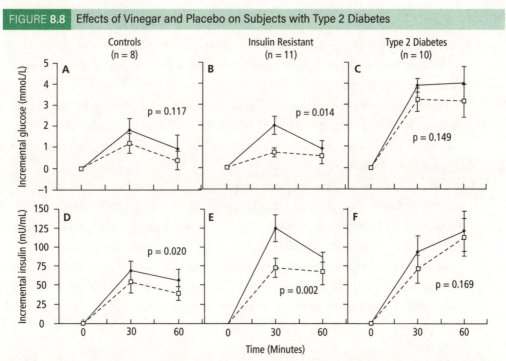

FIGURE 8.8 Effects of Vinegar and Placebo on Subjects with Type 2 Diabetes

Effects of vinegar (□) and placebo (♦) on plasma glucose (A–C) and insulin (D–F) responses after a standard meal in control subjects, insulin-resistant subjects, and subjects with type 2 diabetes. Values are means ± SE. The P values represent a significant effect of treatment (multivariate ANOVA repeated-measures test). © 2004 American Diabetes Association.[126]

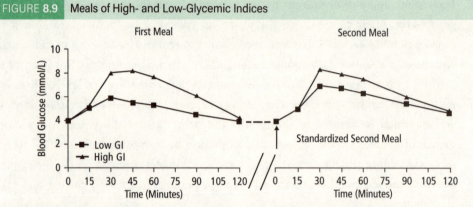

FIGURE 8.9 Meals of High- and Low-Glycemic Indices

Example of blood glucose curves to a first and second meal in response to meals of high- and low-glycemic indices. A meal with a low GI has a lower postprandial glycemic response during the first meal compared with a high-GI meal, and can lower the glycemic response to a standardized second meal. © 2012 J. A. Fletcher et al.[127]

insulin levels, but also helped lower triglyceride levels.[128] A caution with the ingestion of ACV, be sure to dilute it in 6 oz of water, as if taken straight it can damage the enamel on your teeth.

Lemon and lime juice can similarly impact postprandial glucose levels, but not quite as much as ACV. It's worth squeezing between two and four wedges into your water at lunch and dinner and enjoying with your meal, as it has been found to reduce peak glucose spikes by 30%.[129]

8. **Use the second meal effect to your advantage.** This is another great hack that you can use to lower your glucose peak and ensure that you maintain a healthy insulin sensitivity. By eating some carbohydrates, preferably complex carbs from plants, in your first meal, you can "prime" your pancreas to have insulin at the ready for your second meal that contains carbs. This quick insulin release improves glucose uptake by your muscles and liver, reducing the circulating glucose in your bloodstream. This even works overnight, so your meal at dinner with complex, low-glycemic carbs (before 8:00 p.m., right!?) will help you lower your glucose peak at breakfast the next day.[130]

9. **Do very low-intensity exercise after your meal. Go for a walk!** Right after a meal is a great time to go for a walk or do some very low-intensity exercise. Just get moving and do something to help reduce the circulating blood glucose levels. Very low-intensity exercise enhances glucose uptake into the muscles, as muscle contraction serves as a

signal for the protein glucose transporter type 4 (GLUT-4) receptors to shuttle glucose across the cell membrane wall and into the muscle cells.[131] A simple walk can have profound effects on your glucose levels and it's so easy to just go for a 20- to 30-minute walk around the neighborhood, enjoy some sights and fresh air, and also get in some quality time with a loved one. It doesn't need to be a "workout," and intensity should be kept low, with your heart rate between 70 to 80% of your threshold heart rate. See Figure 8.10.

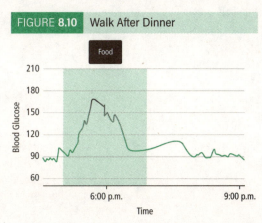

A meal with a glucose peak of 170 was quickly reduced to 90–100 by just going for an easy, 30-minute walk after dinner.

> **CHAPTER 9**

Putting It All Together

MY GOAL IN THIS BOOK has been to take you from newbie in using a continuous glucose monitor (CGM) to being an excellent user of this new technology in training and competing. If your initial feeling about using a CGM was, "I have no idea what these graphs mean, and how I am supposed to understand and interpret them. What am I supposed to change with this information?" then I hope you're well on your way to becoming an advanced user who now is more likely to say, "Hey, check this out: if I eat this sports gel from company X, it doesn't give me much of an increase in glucose, but if I eat this other sports gel from company Y, then it blows me up and gives me a hypo crash. I'd better use the one from company X." I hope that this book will help you with your athletic performance, whether that's just improving at the local pickleball court or at the CrossFit class, or maybe even winning an Olympic Gold Medal. I also hope that you read Chapter 8 again and take to heart the opportunity you have to improve your longevity and vitality. A CGM can make a real difference in your health long-term; it's a great tool to help change your behavior. Please consider checking out my website dedicated to improving your fitness with a CGM and joining my newsletter list: www.Trainingand CompetingwithaCGM.com.

A REVIEW OF THE STEPS

You've read through all the steps to getting started with a CGM, and I've discussed some of the advanced case studies, along with the science behind the responses to different meals, movement, and mood. Now, let's put it all together.

Step 1: Data Collection

Your first step is to collect data. Don't change anything in your current diet for at least two weeks. You need to understand what your current diet, exercise, and moods are doing to your glucose levels without making any changes. It's important that you get a good grasp on what causes your glucose spikes and drops, and how you're creating those. Discovering how you might be on a "slow slide" throughout the afternoon or how you might be creating a reactive hypo crash can be enlightening. Figuring out what your fasted baseline is, along with your pre-meal baseline, will help you to see if that changes over time.

Step 2: Begin to Make Small but Effective Changes

After two weeks, you should begin to make small changes to your diet to see how those impact your glucose responses. Here's where you might change your normal high-glycemic breakfast to something more low-glycemic, simply by adding in some healthy fats like ground flax seeds or organic almond butter. Here's where you should try to do the "food stacking" method I wrote about, along with using some of the glucose hacks to reduce your spikes. You'll also want to begin to change your sports nutrition to see how you can better stabilize your glucose levels over your workout. You should ensure you've the right level of glucose at the start of the workout and, after you finish your workout, replenish your glycogen stores completely, creating just the glucose spike you want.

Step 3: Do Some Testing!

Now you can get serious about testing the limits and begin to learn more about your individual responses. You should do the tests that I outlined in Chapter 3, so that you can learn if you're a fast or slow responder to glucose ingestion. Trying new things here is encouraged. What will happen to your workouts and energy level if you give a whole food, plant-based diet a try for a month or two? What happens when you increase your consumption of proteins before and during your workouts? What does eating later at night do to your nightly average glucose?

Step 4: Learn Your Optimal Glucose Zones

Where do you perform best? What amount of glucose makes you feel strongest and in a good mood to perform? Using the testing data from Step 3, you should be able to learn where you need to keep your glucose for peak training and competing. Remember that you could have multiple glucose zones, especially if you do more than one sport, so factor that into the equation. These are your individual responses for right now. These can, and will, change in the future, especially as the changes you make in Step 2 continue to improve your understanding of glucose. You'll want to retest these zones every 12 weeks or whenever you feel like you've seen a shift in your fasted or pre-meal glucose levels.

Step 5: Interpreting Your Data

This is critical to your improvement. It's vitally important that you spend time each day creating a "range" around your workouts, around your sleep data, and your meals. This way you can

CHAPTER 9: Putting It All Together   151

learn what your glucose averages are, your glucose peaks, and how long your glucose takes to come down from a peak. Here is where you should also track your food intake, and hopefully your CGM app does a good job of helping with this extra task. Look at the graphs throughout your day but also don't obsess over them. Remember that glucose rises are normal and that "keto is *not* the answer!"

Step 6: Training and Competing with Your CGM

To improve your athletic ability, you need to go out, train smart, and put in the hard work. You should now have the knowledge to ensure that you "prime" yourself correctly, keep within your glucose performance zones as you workout or compete, and know exactly how to eat after to create just the glucose response that you want. You'll also learn that in competition, you might just have different responses and outcomes because your epinephrine (adrenaline) heavily impacts your glucose release from stored glycogen. Put yourself in different scenarios and try different glucose strategies. Once you learn what works, stick with it.

Step 7: Use Your CGM to Improve Your Longevity and Vitality

Whether you're 25 or 65, you can make a difference. You can make a difference in your metabolic health even if you've eaten like crap all your life. You have the tools now and the knowledge to change your metabolic health for the better, increase your longevity, and continue to improve as you age. As athletes, we all want to continue to be healthy and live a strong and purposeful lifestyle as we age. Continue to learn and become a student of improving your longevity and vitality. The positive changes will only occur if you're willing to make those changes and stick with them. It could take a year of a major diet change to improve your insulin sensitivity, so don't give up before you give those changes a real chance to work.

SOME FINAL THOUGHTS

While using a CGM can be very exciting and interesting as you learn more and more about yourself and the world around you, be sure to avoid the "obsession" syndrome. Inserting a CGM is easy to do and seeing your responses can be very addictive, so it's important to keep things in perspective as well. Have that ice cream or candy bar if you want it, and don't worry about what your glucose goes to. Just don't make it a daily thing. Choose those special treats, and ensure you use some of the ways to minimize your spike. My personal favorite is tater tots. But, before I have these I take one to two tablespoons of apple cider vinegar, eat a big salad, and put some amla in my water, so that I get to enjoy my guilty pleasure and keep my glucose spike to a minimum.

It's important that you live life to the fullest. Using a CGM should be another powerful tool in your toolbox to improve your athletic performance and not something that takes happiness out of your life. Take breaks from using your CGM and maintain the good habits that you've created. Yes, I know the accountability with using a CGM is also addictive, but trust in your new habit, and your knowledge about how you react. I know that after using a CGM for a year, and learning your responses to every food, mood, and movement, you'll be able to accurately predict your glucose response when you don't have one on. I've found that using a CGM has become so profound for behavior change. It's a tool that can help you to continue to improve and see your hard work paying off, and it can give you the confidence to excel in your sport and reach the top of the podium.

Appendix A

Date	Food Ingested	Glucose Level Before	Glucose Peak	Glucose Average	Time to Return to Pre-Meal Level

Date	Food Ingested	Glucose Level Before	Glucose Peak	Glucose Average	Time to Return to Pre-Meal Level

Date	Food Ingested	Glucose Level Before	Glucose Peak	Glucose Average	Time to Return to Pre-Meal Level

Date	Food Ingested	Glucose Level Before	Glucose Peak	Glucose Average	Time to Return to Pre-Meal Level

Notes

PREFACE

1. Aaron Stevenson, email conversation direct with author, August 2024.

2. "How Blood Vessel Damage from High Glucose Concentrations Unfolds," *ScienceDaily*, June 5, 2019, https://www.sciencedaily.com/releases/2019/06/190605105950.htm.

3. Molly Knudsen, "What Is Metabolic Health, and How Is It Measured?," *mindbodygreen*, July 31, 2023, https://www.mindbodygreen.com/articles/what-is-metabolic-health-and -how-to-tell-if-your-metabolically-healthy?srsltid=AfmBOoqe9HScZlCQtf4GBgLo9fqp MP52hdu3bY9HiGyUrFN4c1VeBQ2-.

4. Jonny Bowden and Stephen Sinatra, *The Great Cholesterol Myth* (Quarto Publishing, 2020), 129–131.

5. Maryanne Demasi et al., "The Cholesterol and Calorie Hypotheses Are Both Dead—It Is Time to Focus on the Real Culprit: Insulin Resistance," *The Pharmaceutical Journal*, July 14, 2017, https://pharmaceutical-journal.com/article/opinion/the-cholesterol-and -calorie-hypotheses-are-both-dead-it-is-time-to-focus-on-the-real-culprit-insulin -resistance.

6. Ding Ding et al., "Physical Activity, Diet Quality, and All-Cause Cardiovascular Disease and Cancer Mortality: A Prospective Study of 346,627 UK Biobank Participants," *British Journal of Sports Medicine* 56, no. 20 (2022), https://doi.org/10.1136/bjsports-2021-105195.

CHAPTER 1

7. Daniel DeSalvo and Bruce Buckingham, "Continuous Glucose Monitoring: Current Use and Future Directions," *Current Diabetes Reports* 13, no. 5 (2013): 657–662, https://doi.org /10.1007/s11892-013-0398-4.

8. Teresa P. Monsod et al., "Do Sensor Glucose Levels Accurately Predict Plasma Glucose Concentrations During Hypoglycemia and Hyperinsulinemia?" *Diabetes Care* 25, no. 5 (2002): 889–93, https://doi.org/10.2337/diacare.25.5.889.

9. Abimbola A. Akintola et al., "Accuracy of Continuous Glucose Monitoring Measurements in Normo-Glycemic Individuals," *PLoS One* 10, no. 10 (2015), https://doi.org/10.1371 /journal.pone.0139973.

10. Günther Schmelzeisen-Redeker et al., "Time Delay of CGM Sensors: Relevance, Causes and Countermeasures," *Journal of Diabetes Science and Technology* 9, no. 5 (2015): 1006–1015, https://doi.org/10.1177/1932296815590154.

11. Giada Acciaroli et al., "Calibration of Minimally Invasive Continuous Glucose Monitoring Sensors: State-of-The-Art and Current Perspectives," *Biosensors* 8, no. 24 (2018), https://doi.org/10.3390/bios8010024; and Udo Hoss and Erwin Satrya Budiman, "Factory-Calibrated Continuous Glucose Sensors: The Science Behind the Technology," *Diabetes Technology & Therapeutics* 19, no. S2 (2017), https://doi.org/10.1089/dia.2017.0025; Amy-Lee Bowler et al., "The Use of Continuous Glucose Monitors in Sport: Possible Applications and Considerations," *International Journal of Sport Nutrition and Exercise Metabolism* 33, no. 2 (2022): 121–132, https://doi.org/10.1123/ijsnem.2022-0139.

12. David Rodbard, "Continuous Glucose Monitoring: A Review of Successes, Challenges, and Opportunities," *Diabetes Technology & Therapeutics* 18, no. S2 (2016): S3–S13, https://doi.org/10.1089/dia.2015.0417.

13. Discussion on glucose levels with Dr. Stephen McGregor, phone interview direct with author, August 12, 2024.

14. Asker Jeukendrup and Michael Gleeson, *Sport Nutrition,* 4th ed. (Human Kinetics Publishers, 2024). Available from: VitalSource Bookshelf.

15. Dr. Andrew R. Coggan (in email exchange with author) August 13, 2024; Coggan et al., "Effect of Endurance Training on Hepatic Glycogenolysis and Gluconeogenesis During Prolonged Exercise in Men," *American Journal of Physiology* 268, no. 3 (1995): E375–E383, https://doi.org/10.1152/ajpendo.1995.268.3.E375.

16. Jeukendrup and Gleeson, *Sport Nutrition*, 98.

17. Ada Maria Vetere, "Functions of Carbohydrates in the Body," *Torrinomedica*, August 8, 2024, https://www.torrinomedica.it/english/dietology/carbohydrates/functions-of-carbohydrates-in-the-body-3.

18. Jeukendrup and Gleeson, *Sport Nutrition*, 214–216.

CHAPTER 2

19. James M. Lattimer and Mark D. Haub, "Effects of Dietary Fiber and Its Components on Metabolic Health," *Nutrients* 2, no. 12 (2010): 1266–89, https://doi.org/10.3390/nu2121266.

20. Lattimer and Haub "Effects of Dietary Fiber," 1266–89.

21. Fiona S. Atkinson et al., "International Tables of Glycemic Index and Glycemic Load Values 2021: A Systematic Review," *The American Journal of Clinical Nutrition* 114, no. 5 (2021): 1625–1632, https://doi.org/10.1093/ajcn/nqab233.

22. Saidur Rahman MD et al., "Role of Insulin in Health and Disease: An Update," *International Journal of Molecular Science* 22, no. 12 (2021): 6403, https://doi.org/10.3390/ijms22126403.

23. Panayota Mitrou et al., "Vinegar Consumption Increases Insulin-Stimulated Glucose Uptake by the Forearm Muscle in Humans with Type 2 Diabetes," *Journal of Diabetes Research* (2015), https://doi.org/10.1155/2015/175204.

24. H. Liljeberg and I. Björck, "Delayed Gastric Emptying Rate May Explain Improved Glycaemia in Healthy Subjects to a Starchy Meal with Added Vinegar," *European Journal of Clinical Nutrition* 52, no. 5 (1998): 368–71, https://doi.org/10.1038/sj.ejcn.1600572.

25. Hannah Seok et al., "Balsamic Vinegar Improves High Fat-Induced Beta Cell Dysfunction via Beta Cell ABCA1," *Diabetes & Metabolism Journal* 36, no. 4 (2012): 275–9, https://doi.org/10.4093/dmj.2012.36.4.275.

26. Ogawa Nobumasa et al., "Acetic Acid Suppresses the Increase in Disaccharidase Activity That Occurs during Culture of Caco-2 Cells," *The Journal of Nutrition* 130, no. 3 (2000): 507–13, https://doi.org/10.1093/jn/130.3.507.

27. Étienne Myette-Côté et al., "A Ketone Monoester Drink Reduces the Glycemic Response to an Oral Glucose Challenge in Individuals with Obesity: A Randomized Trial," *The American Journal of Clinical Nutrition* 110, no. 6 (2019): 1491–1501, https://doi.org/10.1093/ajcn/nqz232.

28. Jennie C. Brand-Miller et al., "Effect of Alcoholic Beverages on Postprandial Glycemia and Insulinemia in Lean, Young, Healthy Adults," *The American Journal of Clinical Nutrition* 85, no. 6 (2007): 1545–51, https://doi.org/10.1093/ajcn/85.6.1545.

29. James H. O'Keefe et al., "Alcohol and Cardiovascular Health: The Razor-Sharp Double-Edged Sword," Journal of the American College of Cardiology 50, no. 11 (2007): 1009–14, https://doi.org/10.1016/j.jacc.2007.04.089.

30. Peter Attia, "Is Low-to-Moderate Alcohol Consumption Beneficial for Longevity?," *Peter Attia–MD*, January 3, 2024, https://peterattiamd.com/low-to-moderate-alcohol-consumption-and-longevity; "No Level of Alcohol Consumption Is Safe for Our Health," *World Health Organization*, January 4, 2024, https://www.who.int/europe/news/item/04-01-2023-no-level-of-alcohol-consumption-is-safe-for-our-health; Michael Le Page, "Why Many Studies Wrongly Claim It's Healthy to Drink a Little Alcohol," *NewScientist*, July 25, 2024, https://www.newscientist.com/article/2441154-why-many-studies-wrongly-claim-its-healthy-to-drink-a-little-alcohol.

CHAPTER 3

31. Thomas K. Mathew et al., "Blood Glucose Monitoring" in *StatPearls [Internet]* (Treasure Island (FL): StatPearls Publishing), last updated April 23, 2023, https://www.ncbi.nlm.nih.gov/books/NBK555976.

32. Kristina Skroce et al., "Real World Interstitial Glucose Profiles of a Large Cohort of Physically Active Men and Women," *Sensors* 23, no. 3 (2024): 744, https://doi.org/10.3390/s24030744.

33. Skroce, "Real World Interstitial Glucose Profiles," 744.

34. Ciara Morris et al., "Identification of Differential Responses to an Oral Glucose Tolerance Test in Healthy Adults," *PLoS One* 8, no. 8 (2013): e72890, https://doi.org/10.1371/journal.pone.0072890.

35. Skroce, "Real World Interstitial Glucose Profiles," 744.

36. Kotone Tanaka, "Fasting Biochemical Hypoglycemia and Related-Factors in Non-Diabetic Population: Kanagawa Investigation of Total Check-up Data from National Database-8," *World Journal of Diabetes* 12, no. 7 (2021): 1131–1140, https://doi.org/10.4239/wjd.v12.i7.1131.

CHAPTER 4

37. Charlie Cawsey, "A Guide to Understanding the Pizza Effect in Diabetes" *Type One Style*, February 6, 2023, https://www.typeonestyle.com/en-us/blogs/guide-key-strategies-to-improve-mental-health-for-people-with-type-one-diabetes/a-guide-to-understanding-the-pizza-effect-in-diabetes.

38. Anne Smith et al., *Wardlaw's Contemporary Nutrition*, 12th ed. (McGraw Hill, 2015), 429.

39. Milou Beelen et al., "Nutritional Strategies to Promote Postexercise Recovery," *International Journal of Sport Nutrition and Exercise Metabolism* 20, no. 6 (2010): 515–32, https://doi.org/10.1123/ijsnem.20.6.515.

40. Jeffrey A. Rothschild et al., "What Should I Eat Before Exercise? Pre-Exercise Nutrition and the Response to Endurance Exercise: Current Prospective and Future Directions," *Nutrients* 12, no. 11 (2020): 3473, https://doi.org/10.3390/nu12113473.

41. Asker Jeukendrup, "A Step Towards Personalized Sports Nutrition: Carbohydrate Intake During Exercise," *Sports Medicine* 44 (2014): 25–33, https://doi.org/10.1007/s40279-014-0148-z.

42. Asker Jeukendrup and Sophie Killer, "The Myths Surrounding Pre-Exercise Carbohydrate Feeding," *Annals of Nutrition & Metabolism* 57, no. 2 (2011): 18–25, https://doi.org/10.1159/000322698.

43. Asker Jeukendrup, "What to Eat the Hour Before a Race?," accessed January 27, 2025, https://www.mysportscience.com/post/2015/02/05/what-to-eat-the-hour-before-a-race.

44. Trent Stellingwerff and Gregory R. Cox, "Systematic Review: Carbohydrate Supplementation on Exercise Performance or Capacity of Varying Durations," *Applied Physiology, Nutrition, and Metabolism* 39, no. 9 (2014): 998–1011, https://doi.org/10.1139/apnm-2014-0027.

45. Asker Jeukendrup, "A Step Towards Personalized Sports Nutrition: Carbohydrate Intake During Exercise," *Sports Medicine* 44 (2014): 25–33, https://doi.org/10.1007/s40279-014-0148-z.

46. Samuel A. Levine et al., "Some Changes in the Chemical Constituents of the Blood Following a Marathon Race," *Journal of the American Medical Association* 82, no. 22 (1924): 1778–79, https://doi.org/10.1001/jama.1924.02650480034015.

47. Kristina Skroce et al., "Real World Interstitial Glucose Profiles of a Large Cohort of Physically Active Men and Women," *Sensors* 24, no. 3 (2024): 744, https://doi.org/10.3390/s24030744.

48. Dr. Andrew R. Coggan, email conversation with author, August 5, 2024. Heart rate is under the control of both the parasympathetic and sympathetic nervous systems.

    The latter also contributes to the regulation of hepatic glucose production, mostly indirectly by regulating (suppressing) insulin secretion (thus relieving the inhibitory effect of insulin, but secondarily/directly (at higher degrees of sympathetic activation) by stimulating hepatic glycogenolysis and gluconeogenesis. In other words, both elevations in heart rate and in glucose production would be *consequences* of SNS activation (vs. high heart rate *causing* an increase).

49. Asker Jeukendrup and Michael Gleeson, *Sport Nutrition*, 4th ed. (Human Kinetics Publishers, 2024), 443.

50. Chris Poole et al., "The Role of Post-Exercise Nutrient Administration on Muscle Protein Synthesis and Glycogen Synthesis," *Journal of Sports Science and Medicine* 9, no. 3 (2010): 354–63, https://pmc.ncbi.nlm.nih.gov/articles/PMC3761704; David S. Rowlands et al., "Protein-Leucine Fed Dose Effects on Muscle Protein Synthesis After Endurance Exercise," *Medicine & Science in Sports & Exercise* 47, no. 3 (2015): 547–55, https://doi.org/10.1249/MSS.0000000000000447.

51. Monique Ryan, email message to author, August 6, 2024.

CHAPTER 5

52. "About the Stability Score," Levels website, accessed January 27, 2025, https://support.levels.com/article/266-about-the-stability-score-feature.

53. Concepción Peiró et al., "Inflammation, Glucose, and Vascular Cell Damage: The Role of the Pentose Phosphate Pathway," *Cardiovascular Diabetology* 15, no. 82 (2016), https://doi.org/10.1186/s12933-016-0397-2 (erratum in: *Cardiovascular Diabetology* 16, no. 25 (2017), https://doi.org/10.1186/s12933-017-0502-1); Nuria Lafuente et al., "The Deleterious Effect of High Concentrations of D-Glucose Requires Pro-Inflammatory Preconditioning," *Journal of Hypertension* 26, no. 3 (2008): 478–85, https://doi.org/10.1097/HJH.0b013e3282f331fb.

54. Justin B. Echouffo-Tcheugui et al., "Diagnosis and Management of Prediabetes: A Review," *Journal of American Medical Association* 329, no. 14 (2023): 1206–1216, https://doi.org/10.1001/jama.2023.4063; Laura Mayans, "Metabolic Syndrome: Insulin Resistance and Prediabetes," *FP Essentials* 435 (2015): 11–6, https://pubmed.ncbi.nlm.nih.gov/26280340.

55. Asker Jeukendrup and Michael Gleeson, *Sport Nutrition*, 4th ed. (Human Kinetics Publishers, 2024), 105. Available from: VitalSource Bookshelf.

CHAPTER 6

56. Tracey J. Smith, "Interstitial Glucose Concentrations and Hypoglycemia During 2 Days of Caloric Deficit and Sustained Exercise: A Double-Blind, Placebo-Controlled Trial," *Journal of Applied Physiology* 121, no. 5 (2016): 1208–1216, https://doi.org/10.1152/japplphysiol.00432.2016.

57. Alexandra M. Coates et al., "Overreached Endurance Athletes Demonstrate Alterations in Exercising Carbohydrate Utilization Applicable to Training Monitoring," August 25, 2023, https://doi.org/10.51224/SRXIV.321.

58. Asker E. Jeukendrup and Sophie C. Killer, "The Myths Surrounding Pre-Exercise Carbohydrate Feeding" *Annals of Nutrition & Metabolism* 57, no. 2 (2011): 18–25, https://doi.org/10.1159/000322698.

59. M. A. Van Nieuwenhoven et al., "Gastrointestinal Function During Exercise: Comparison of Water, Sports Drink, and Sports Drink with Caffeine," *Journal of Applied Physiology* 89, no. 3 (2000):1079–85, https://doi.org/10.1152/jappl.2000.89.3.1079.

60. Sophie E. Yeo et al., "Caffeine Increases Exogenous Carbohydrate Oxidation During Exercise," *Journal of Applied Physiology* 99, no. 3 (2005): 844–50, https://doi.org/10.1152/japplphysiol.00170.2005.

61. University of Warwick, "How Blood Vessel Damage from High Glucose Concentrations Unfolds," *ScienceDaily*, June 5, 2019, www.sciencedaily.com/releases/2019/06/190605105950.htm.

62. K. M. Zawadzki et al., "Carbohydrate-Protein Complex Increases the Rate of Muscle Glycogen Storage After Exercise," *Journal of Applied Physiology* 72, no. 5 (1992): 1854–59, https://doi.org/10.1152/jappl.1992.72.5.1854.

63. "Animal Protein and Cancer Risk," Osher Center for Integrative Health (University of California San Francisco), accessed January 27, 2025, https://osher.ucsf.edu/patient-care/integrative-medicine-resources/cancer-and-nutrition/faq/animal-protein-cancer-risk.

64. Matthew Budoff et al., "Carbohydrate Restriction-Induced Elevations in LDL-Cholesterol and Atherosclerosis: The KETO Trial," *JACC Advances* 3, no. 8 (2024): 101109, https://doi.org/10.1016/j.jacadv.2024.101109.

65. R. S. Sherwin and L. Saccà, "Effect of Epinephrine on Glucose Metabolism in Humans: Contribution of the Liver," *American Journal of Physiology* 247, no. 2 (1984): E157–65, https://doi.org/10.1152/ajpendo.1984.247.2.E157.

CHAPTER 7

66. Jessica Lucier and Priyanka M. Mathias, "Type 1 Diabetes" in *StatPearls [Internet]* (Treasure Island (FL): StatPearls Publishing), last updated October 5, 2024, https://www.ncbi.nlm.nih.gov/books/NBK507713.

67. Dr. Michael Riddell (professor at York University) in discussion with the author, August 27, 2024.

68. Phil Southerland, founder of Supersapiens and Team Type 1, in discussion with the author, August 13, 2024.

69. Phil Bartels (type 1 athlete coach) in discussion with the author, August 14, 2024.

70. Dessi P. Zaharieva et al., "Improved Open-Loop Glucose Control with Basal Insulin Reduction 90 Minutes Before Aerobic Exercise in Patients with Type 1 Diabetes on Continuous Subcutaneous Insulin Infusion," *Diabetes Care* 42, no. 5 (2019): 824–831, https://doi.org/10.2337/dc18-2204.

71. Asker Jeukendrup and Michael Gleeson, *Sport Nutrition*, 4th ed. (Human Kinetics Publishers, 2024).

72. Sam N. Scott et al., "Post-Exercise Recovery for the Endurance Athlete with Type 1 Diabetes: A Consensus Statement," *The Lancet Diabetes & Endocrinology* 9, no. 5 (2021): 304–317, https://doi.org/10.1016/s2213-8587(21)00054-1.

73. M. J. MacDonald, "Postexercise Late-Onset Hypoglycemia in Insulin-Dependent Diabetic Patients," *Diabetes Care* 10, no. 5 (1987): 584–588, https://doi.org/10.2337/diacare.10.5.584.

74. Othmar Moser et al., "Glucose Management for Exercise Using Continuous Glucose Monitoring (CGM) and Intermittently Scanned CGM (isCGM) Systems in Type 1 Diabetes: Position Statement of the European Association for the Study of Diabetes (EASD) and of the International Society for Pediatric and Adolescent Diabetes (ISPAD) Endorsed by JDRF and Supported by the American Diabetes Association (ADA)," *Diabetologia* 63 (2020): 2501–2520, https://doi.org/10.1007/s00125-020-05263-9.

75. Michael C. Riddell et al., "Exercise Management in Type 1 Diabetes: A Consensus Statement," *The Lancet Diabetes & Endocrinology* 5, no. 5 (2017): 377–390, https://doi.org/10.1016/S2213-8587(17)30014-1.

76. "Hyperglycemia (High Blood Glucose)," American Diabetes Association, accessed January 29, 2025, https://diabetes.org/living-with-diabetes/treatment-care/hyperglycemia.

77. Phil Bartels discussion, August 14, 2024.

78. Roy Jentjens and Asker E. Jeukendrup, "Determinants of Post-Exercise Glycogen Synthesis During Short-Term Recovery," *Sports Medicine* 33 (2003): 117–44, https://doi.org/10.2165/00007256-200333020-00004; J. L. Ivy and C. H. Kuo, "Regulation of GLUT4 Protein and Glycogen Synthase During Muscle Glycogen Synthesis After Exercise," *Acta Physiologica Scandinavica* 162, no. 3 (1998): 295–304, https://doi.org/10.1046/j.1365-201X.1998.0302e.x.

79. Hugh H. K. Fullagar, "Sleep and Recovery in Team Sport: Current Sleep," *International Journal of Sports Physiology Performance* 10, no. 8 (2015): 950–57, https://doi.org/10.1123/ijspp.2014-0565.

80. Phil Bartels discussion, August 14, 2024.

81. "Blood Sugar & Stress in Diabetes," University of California San Francisco, Diabetes Teaching Center, accessed January 29, 2025, https://diabetesteachingcenter.ucsf.edu/blood-glucose-stress-diabetes.

82. Phil Bartels, email message to author, September 3, 2024.

83. Cyrus Khambatta and Robby Barbaro, *Mastering Diabetes* (Penguin Random House, 2020).

84. Emily Eyth and Roopa Naik, "Hemoglobin A1C" in *StatPearls [Internet]* (Treasure Island (FL): StatPearls Publishing, 2024), last updated March 13, 2023,: https://www.ncbi.nlm.nih.gov/books/NBK549816.

85. "eAG/A1C Conversion Calculator," American Diabetes Association, accessed January 29, 2025, https://professional.diabetes.org/glucose_calc.

86. A Gonzalez et al., "Impact of Mismatches in HbA_{1c} vs Glucose Values on the Diagnostic Classification of Diabetes and Prediabetes," *Diabetic Medicine* 37, no. 4 (2020): 689–696, https://doi.org/10.1111/dme.14181.

87. Kristina Skroce, email message to author, September 19, 2024.

CHAPTER 8

88. "Causes of Insulin Resistance: The Personal Fat Threshold," Nourished by Science, published September 6, 2023, https://nourishedbyscience.com/personal-fat-threshold.

89. Nourished by Science, "Causes of Insulin Resistance: The Personal Fat Threshold."

90. B. Ahrén, "Glucose: Glucose Tolerance" in *The Encyclopedia of Human Nutrition*, ed. Benjamin Caballero, 3rd ed (Academic Press, 2013), 381–386, https://doi.org/10.1016/B978-0-12-375083-9.00134-3.

91. Seung-Hwan Lee et al., "Potentiation of the Early-Phase Insulin Response by a Prior Meal Contributes to the Second-Meal Phenomenon in Type 2 Diabetes," *American Journal of Physiology-Endocrinology and Metabolism* 301, no. 5 (2011): E984–E990, https://doi.org/10.1152/ajpendo.00244.2011.

92. Furio Brighenti, "Colonic Fermentation of Indigestible Carbohydrates Contributes to the Second-Meal Effect," *The American Journal of Clinical Nutrition* 83, no. 4 (2006): 817–822, https://doi.org/10.1093/ajcn/83.4.817.

93. Steven Daniel Funk et al., "Hyperglycemia and Endothelial Dysfunction in Atherosclerosis: Lessons from Type 1 Diabetes," *International Journal of Vascular Medicine* (2012), https://doi.org/10.1155/2012/569654.

94. Funk, "Hyperglycemia and Endothelial Dysfunction."

95. Malgorzata Teodorowicz, "Immunomodulation by Processed Animal Feed: The Role of Maillard Reaction Products and Advanced Glycation End-Products (AGEs)," *Frontiers in Immunology* 9 (2018), https://doi.org/10.3389/fimmu.2018.02088; Izabela Sadowska-Bartosz and Grzegorz Bartosz, "Effect of Glycation Inhibitors on Aging and Age-Related Diseases," *Mechanisms of Ageing and Development* 160 (2016): 1–18, https://doi.org/10.1016/j.mad.2016.09.006.

96. Michael Greger, *How Not to Age* (Flatiron Books, 2023), 55.

97. Alexander Fedintsev and Alexey Moskalev, "Stochastic Non-Enzymatic Modification of Long-Lived Macromolecules—A Missing Hallmark of Aging," *Ageing Research Reviews* 62 (2020), https://doi.org/10.1016/j.arr.2020.101097.

98. Arianna Bettiga et al., "The Modern Western Diet Rich in Advanced Glycation End-Products (AGES): An Overview of its Impact on Obesity and Early Progression of Renal Pathology," *Nutrients* 11, no. 8 (2019): 1748, https://doi.org/10.3390/nu11081748.

99. M. E. Garay-Sevilla et al., "The Potential Role of Dietary Advanced Glycation Endproducts in the Development of Chronic Non-Infectious Diseases: A Narrative Review," *Nutrition Research Reviews* 33, no. 2 (2020): 298–311, https://doi.org/10.1017/S0954422420000104.

100. Jie-Hua Chen et al., "Role of Advanced Glycation End Products in Mobility and Considerations in Possible Dietary and Nutritional Intervention Strategies," *Nutrition & Metabolism* 15, no. 72 (2018), https://doi.org/10.1186/s12986-018-0306-7.

101. Chandan Prasad et al., "Advanced Glycation End Products and Risks for Chronic Diseases: Intervening Through Lifestyle Modification," *American Journal of Lifestyle Medicine* 13, no. 4 (2017): 384–404, https://doi.org/10.1177/1559827617708991.

102. Jamie Uribarri et al., "Advanced Glycation End Products in Foods and a Practical Guide to Their Reduction in the Diet," *Journal of the Academy of Nutrition and Dietetics* 110, no. 6 (2010): 911–916.E12, https://doi.org/10.1016/j.jada.2010.03.018.

103. Uribarri, "Advanced Glycation End Products," 911–916.E12.

104. Dr. Michael Greger, "What to Eat to Live Longer: Ageing Expert Dr Michael Greger Reveals His Definitive Guide to the Foods That Will Dial Down Your 'Grim Reaper Gene,'" *Daily Mail*, February 2, 2024, https://www.dailymail.co.uk/health/article-13038429/ageing-DR-MICHAEL-GREGER-diet-live-longer.html; Wiramon Rungratanawanich et al.,

"Advanced Glycation End Products (AGEs) and Other Adducts in Aging-Related Diseases and Alcohol-Mediated Tissue Injury," *Experimental & Molecular Medicine* 53, no. 2 (2021): 168–88, http://doi.org/10.1038/s12276-021-00561-7.

105. Michael Greger and Gene Stone, *How Not to Die* (Macmillan, 2016).

106. Uribarri, "Advanced Glycation End Products," 911–916.E12.

107. Miwako Tsunosue et al., "An A-Glucosidase Inhibitor, Acarbose Treatment Decreases Serum Levels of Glyceraldehyde-Derived Advanced Glycation End Products (AGEs) in Patients with Type 2 Diabetes," *Clinical and Experimental Medicine* 10, no. 2 (2010): 139–41, https://doi.org/10.1007/s10238-009-0074-9.

108. Threshold heart rate is the highest average heart rate you can maintain for roughly 30–60 minutes.

109. François Mariotti and Christopher D. Gardner, "Dietary Protein and Amino Acids in Vegetarian Diets—A Review," *Nutrients* 11, no. 11 (2019): 2661, https://doi.org/10.3390/nu11112661.

110. V. R. Young and P. L. Pellett, "Plant Proteins in Relation to Human Protein and Amino Acid Nutrition," *American Journal of Clinical Nutrition* 59, no. 5 (1994): 1203S–1212S, https://doi.org/10.1093/ajcn/59.5.1203S.

111. Mark F. McCarty, "GCN2 and FGF21 are Likely Mediators of the Protection from Cancer, Autoimmunity, Obesity, and Diabetes Afforded by Vegan Diets," *Medical Hypotheses* 83, no. 3 (2014): 365–71, https://doi.org/10.1016/j.mehy.2014.06.014; Barbara C. Halpern et al., "The Effect of Replacement of Methionine by Homocystine on Survival of Malignant and Normal Adult Mammalian Cells in Culture," *Proceedings of the National Academy of Sciences* 71, no. 4 (1974): 1133–6, https://doi.org/10.1073/pnas.71.4.1133.

112. Maria Cristina Ruiz et al., "Protein Methionine Content and MDA-lysine Adducts Are Inversely Related to Maximum Life Span in the Heart of Mammals," *Mechanisms of Ageing and Development* 126, no. 10 (2005): 1106–14, https://doi.org/10.1016/j.mad.2005.04.005.

113. Ioannis Delimaris, "Adverse Effects Associated with Protein Intake Above the Recommended Dietary Allowance for Adults," *International Scholarly Research Notices* (2013): 126929, https://doi.org/10.5402/2013/126929.

114. Monica H. Carlsen et al., "The Total Antioxidant Content of More Than 3100 Foods, Beverages, Spices, Herbs and Supplements Used Worldwide," *Nutrition Journal* 9, no. 3 (2010), https://doi.org/10.1186/1475-2891-9-3.

115. Pankaj Pathak et al., "The Effect of *Emblica Officinalis* Diet on Lifespan, Sexual Behavior, and Fitness Characters in Drosophila Melanogaster," *An International Quarterly Journal of Research in Ayurveda* 32, no. 2 (2011): 279–84, https://doi.org/10.4103/0974-8520.92544.

116. Muhammad Shoaib Akhtar et al., "Effect of Amla Fruit (*Emblica Officinalis Gaertn.*) on Blood Glucose and Lipid Profile of Normal Subjects and Type 2 Diabetic Patients," *International Journal of Food Sciences Nutrition* 62, no. 6 (2011): 609–16, https://doi.org/10.3109/09637486.2011.560565.

117. Mahendra Parkash Kapoor et al., "Clinical Evaluation of *Emblica Officinalis Gatertn* (Amla) in Healthy Human Subjects: Health Benefits and Safety Results from a Randomized, Double-Blind, Crossover Placebo-Controlled Study," *Contemporary Clinical Trials Communications* 17 (2020): 100499, https://doi.org/10.1016/j.conctc.2019.100499.

118. Pingali Usharani et al., "Evaluation of the Effects of a Standardized Aqueous Extract of *Phyllanthus Emblica* Fruits on Endothelial Dysfunction, Oxidative Stress, Systemic Inflammation and Lipid Profile in Subjects with Metabolic Syndrome: A Randomised, Double Blind, Placebo Controlled Clinical Study," *BMC Complementary Medicine and Therapies* 19, no. 97 (2019), https://doi.org/10.1186/s12906-019-2509-5.

119. Muhammad Shoaib Akhtar, "Effect of Amla Fruit," 609–16.

120. Paul Holvoet et al., "Oxidized LDL and Malondialdehyde-Modified LDL in Patients with Acute Coronary Syndromes and Stable Coronary Artery Disease," *Circulation* 98, no. 15 (1998): 1487–94, https://doi.org/10.1161/01.cir.98.15.1487.

121. George Henderson et al., "Linoleic Acid and Diabetes Prevention," *The Lancet Diabetes & Endocrinology* 6, no. 1 (2018): 12–13, https://doi.org/10.1016/s2213-8587(17)30404-7.

122. Monica L. Bertoia et al., "Changes in Intake of Fruits and Vegetables and Weight Change in United States Men and Women Followed for up to 24 Years: Analysis from Three Prospective Cohort Studies," *PLOS Medicine* 12, no. 9 (2015), https://doi.org/10.1371/journal.pmed.1001878.

123. Ding Ding et al., "Physical Activity, Diet Quality and All-Cause Cardiovascular Disease and Cancer Mortality: A Prospective Study of 346 627 UK Biobank Participants," *British Journal of Sports Medicine* 56, no. 20 (2022): 1148–1156, https://doi.org/10.1136/bjsports-2021-105195.

124. Carol S. Johnston et al., "Vinegar Improves Insulin Sensitivity to a High-Carbohydrate Meal in Subjects with Insulin Resistance or Type 2 Diabetes," *Diabetes Care* 27, no. 1 (2004): 281–282, https://doi.org/10.2337/diacare.27.1.281.

125. Carol. S. Johnston et al., "Preliminary Evidence That Regular Vinegar Ingestion Favorably Influences Hemoglobin A1c Values in Individuals with Type 2 Diabetes Mellitus," *Diabetes Research and Clinical Practice* 84, no. 2 (2009): e15–e17, https://doi.org/10.1016/j.diabres.2009.02.005.

126. American Diabetes Association, *Vinegar Improves Insulin Sensitivity to a High-Carbohydrate Meal in Subjects With Insulin Resistance or Type 2 Diabetes* (American Diabetes Association, 2004). Copyright and all rights reserved. Material from this publication has been used with the permission of American Diabetes Association.

127. Justin A. Fletcher et al., "The Second Meal Effect and Its Influence on Glycemia," *Journal of Nutritional Disorders & Therapy.* 2, no. 1 (2012): 108, https://doi.org/10.4172/2161-0509.1000108

128. Panayota Mitrou et al., "Vinegar Consumption Increases Insulin-Stimulated Glucose Uptake by the Forearm Muscle in Humans with Type 2 Diabetes," *Journal of Diabetes Research* (2015) :175204, https://doi.org/10.1155/2015/175204.

129. Daniela Freitas et al., "Lemon Juice, but Not Tea, Reduces the Glycemic Response to Bread in Healthy Volunteers: A Randomized Crossover Trial," *European Journal of Nutrition* 60 (2021): 113–122, https://doi.org/10.1007/s00394-020-02228-x.

130. T. M. Wolever et al., "Second-Meal Effect: Low-Glycemic-Index Foods Eaten at Dinner Improve Subsequent Breakfast Glycemic Response," *American Journal of Clinical Nutrition* 48, no. 4 (1988): 1041–7, https://doi.org/10.1093/ajcn/48.4.1041.

131. Laurie J. Goodyear and Barbara B. Kahn, "Exercise, Glucose Transport, and Insulin Sensitivity," *Annual Review of Medicine* 49 (1998): 235–61, https://doi.org/10.1146/annurev.med.49.1.235.

Glossary

adenosine triphosphate (ATP)   a product of the glycosis process which functions as the "energy currency" of the cell

adipose tissue   technical term for "body fat;" fat cells in the body functioning as energy storage

adrenalin (epinephrine)   Chemical produced as part of the "fight or flight" nervous system response that provokes a glucose spike so the body has energy

advanced glycation end products (AGEs)   Products of the glycation process which are one of the main factors contributing to the ageing process by increasing inflammation and tissue stiffening

alpha-amylase   Secretion of the mouth which slows down starch digestion and increase glucose uptake

amino acids   Chemical that forms the main components of protein. Bodies need a variety, which is achieved by eating a varied diet.

amla powder   Indian Gooseberry, a powerful anti-inflammatory antioxidant

artherosclerosis   build-up of fats and cholesterol on artery walls

beta cells   produced by the pancreas to produce insulin

beta thalassemia   condition in which people have smaller than normal red blood cells

calibration   process of checking CGM monitor data against other sources of data

catabolic functions   metabolic process that breaks down complex molecules into simpler ones

catecholamines   neurotransmitters and hormones that are involved in stress response and can cause gluconeogenesis

complex carbohydrates   carbohydrates with long chains of sugar molecules which take longer to digest and provide more stable blood glucose levels than simple carbohydrates *See also* polysaccharides

cortisol   hormone produced under stressful conditions which has a role in blood glucose regulation

cytokines   part of the immune system which in type 2 diabetes can make cells become more insulin resistant

diabetic ketoacidosis (DKA) condition in which the body begins to break down fat for energy leading to high ketone levels and acidic blood

endothelial cells single cell layer on the inside of all blood vessels which regulate exchanges between bloodstream and tissues

epinephrine *see* adrenalin

fiber bulky element of food that promotes satiety and slows digestion

flavin adenine dinucleotide (FADH2) crucial enzyme in metabolic processes, part of Krebs Cycle

fructose simple sugar coming from natural sources such as fruit, vegetables and honey

gastric emptying rate speed at which the stomach empties contents into the small intestine. Too fast is harmful to the body

glucagon hormone produced by the pancreas which tells the liver to release glycogen stores

glucagon-like peptide 1 (GLP-1) drugs hormone used as a type 2 diabetes medication

gluconeogenesis process by which the liver creates glucose for usage

glucose simple sugar which forms the body's main source of energy and can be stored as glycogen

glucose performance zone (GPZ) range of blood glucose levels where an athlete feels and performs best

glucose tolerance ability of the body to dispose of glucose into cells and tissues after ingestion

GLUT-4 (glucose transporter type 4) glucose transporter in muscle and tissue which shuttles glucose across the cell membrane

Glycation binding of sugar molecules to proteins. *See also* advanced glycation end products (AGEs)

Glycemic Index (GI) foods are categorized as "high," "medium," or "low" GI according to the rate at which they raise blood glucose compared to a reference value

glycogen form of glucose stored in the liver

glycogenesis process of converting excess blood glucose into glycogen

glycogenolysis process of breaking down stored glycogen into glucose so that it can be released for energy purposes

glycolysis energy-producing process in cells which converts glucose into pyruvate and adenosine triphosphate (ATP)

gut microbiome ecosystem of microbes in the intestine which has an impact on blood glucose response

hemoglobin (HbA1c) hemoglobin is a protein in red blood cells that carries oxygen. The HbA1c test measures percentage of red blood cells that have sugar attached to them

Glossary 171

homeostasis narrow range where blood glucose is optimal and which your body will try to return to

hyperglycemia an excess of glucose in the blood which can lead to serious complications if not addressed

hyperinsulinemia elevated insulin levels produced by pancreas

hyperplasia storage of fat in the body as new molecules of fat

hypoglycemia blood glucose levels which are too low. Symptoms include shakiness and confusion and can become serious if unaddressed

indigestible carbohydrates includes soluble and insoluble **fiber** as well as resistant starches. They contribute to the "second meal effect"

inflammation biological response to harmful stimuli in the body

insulin hormone produced by the pancreas which enables glucose to enter cells to provide energy

interstitial glucose measurement method of measuring glucose levels which involves inserting a sensor under the skin

ketoacidosis *see* diabetic ketoacidosis (DKA)

ketones acids made by the body when it breaks down fat for energy purposes in the absence of glucose

Krebs Cycle part of the process through which glucose is turned into energy in cells

leucine amino acid used by skeletal muscle to give energy during exercise

linoleic acid essential omega-6 PUFA which can contribute to **atherosclerosis**

lipogenesis process by which fats ingested alongside carbohydrates are stored

lipolysis metabolic process which enables fats to be used for energy

metabolic health **glucose tolerance** and **insulin** sensitivity are measures of metabolic health

methionine amino acid primarily found in animal proteins

monocytes white blood cells that contribute to "self-preservative" insulin resistance

nicotinamide adenine dinucleotide (NADH) an energy-carrying molecule produced by **glycosis**

oxidative phosphorylation (electron transport chain) part of the process through which glucose is turned into energy in cells

pancreas organ which plays a key role in digestion by producing enzymes including **insulin**

plaque fatty deposit on a blood vessel wall

polysaccharides long-chain carbohydrate made up of smaller carbohydrates (monosaccharides)

preadipocytes cells in waiting which can become fat cells if existing fat cells become saturated

PUFAs (polyunsaturated fatty acids) found in processed food these are thought to play a role in artherosclerosis

Pyruvate   molecule involved in metabolic processes including glycolysis

RAGE (receptors for advanced glycation end products)   when triggered can set off a harmful inflammatory cascade

reactive hypoglycemic crashes   depletion in levels of blood glucose that happen after ingesting carbs

retrogradation   starchy food that has been allowed to cool to convert starch to resistant starch

simple carbohydrates   short chains of basic sugar molecules, including fructose and glucose

subcutaneous fat   body fat stored under the skin

triglycerides   form of stored fat which can be measured as an indicator of metabolic health

type 1 diabetes   condition in which the pancreas produces little to no insulin meaning the individual has to rely on external insulin administration to manage blood glucose

type 2 diabetes   condition whereby the body becomes resistant to insulin and requires careful dietary management and sometimes medication to control blood glucose

visceral fat   stored in cells deep in the body

Index

Abbott's Libre Sense Glucose Sport Biosensor, xi, 2, 6
Acarbose, 137, 145
acetic acid, 28, 30, 145
adenosine triphosphate (ATP), 8, 9–10, 56
adipose tissue, 11, 15, 82, 91, 130
adrenalin (epinephrine), 14, 41, 84, 104, 107, 120
advanced glycation end products (AGEs), 136–137
alcohol, 31
algorithms, 2, 77, 82
alpha-amylase action, 145
amino acids, 71, 140
amla powder, 142–143
animal-derived proteins, 91, 103, 104, 125, 137, 140, 144
apple cider vinegar, 28, 30, 145–146
apps, 5–6, 141
average glucose, 75–76, 123

Barbaro, Robby, 122
Bartels, Phil, 113, 117, 118, 120
baseline glucose, xiv, 34–35, 61, 80, 84–85, 91–92, 127, 133
batteries, 4
Beelen, Milou, 50
Beltran, Michelle, 107–108
beta cells, 11, 28, 112, 122, 135
beta thalassemia, 122
blood glucose, definition, 6–9
blood glucose spikes. *See* glucose spikes
body weight: carbs/protein calculations, 71; obesity, 130, 131; weight gain, 120–122, 127
"bonking," 6–7, 24, 61, 86. *See also* hypoglycemia
brain reliance on glucose, 10, 12
branched cluster dextrin (HBCD), 55

breakfast, 25, 26, 38, 62–63, 70, 107, 134, 146
"buckets," 77

calibration of monitor, 2–3
calorie deficit, 75, 123
carbo loading, 82
catabolic functions, 19
catecholamines, 114. *See also* adrenalin (epinephrine)
cholesterol, 135
citric acid, 30
cliff, 61–62
Coggan, Andrew R., 8, 82
Cohen, Scott, 69
complex carbohydrates, 18–22, 55, 61, 81
cooking foods, 21, 137
cooling foods, 134, 141–142
correlations, vii
cortisol, 120
Cronometer, 141
cytokines, 130

data gathering, 33–34, 44, 149–150
data transfer, 4
deltaG ®, 30–31
desserts, 38
Dexcom G7, 3
diabetes. *See* type 1 diabetes; type 2 diabetes
diabetic coma, 12
diabetic ketoacidosis (DKA), 11, 112, 117
dinner, 38
"double bump" (biphasic spike), 49

early morning exercise, 69, 78, 95
early phase insulin response, 134

eating while exercising, 62, 95–96. *See also* gels; gummies
ectopic fat, 131
Elder, Lorenzo, 51, 68–69
endothelial cells, 101, 135
endurance sports, 56, 62, 67, 71, 87, 116
epinephrine. *See* adrenalin (epinephrine)
epithelial layer, xvi
events (in apps), 33, 37

fast responders, 42, 44, 52–53, 54, 90–91
fasting glucose rate, 35, 80, 94–95, 98, 107
fatigue, 45, 70, 82
fats. *See also* keto diet: as fuel, 10; and glucose levels, 30, 101; Glycemic Index (GI), 22; insulin, 11, 80; recovery phases, 73; type 2 diabetes, 36, 125, 132
fatty acids, 130, 131, 134
fiber, 18, 21, 55, 73, 81, 101, 134, 138
finger-stick glucometers, 1, 2–3, 80
flavin adenine dinucleotide (FADH2), 10
Food and Drug Administration (FDA), xi, 5, 6
food stacking, 27–28, 141, 150
fructose, 14, 18, 42, 53, 88
Functional Threshold Tests (FTP), 57, 72

Gasperini, Peter, 56–58
gastric emptying rate, 28, 55, 60, 73, 80
gels, 24–26, 39–41, 52–53, 58, 61–62, 87–88, 95–96
Gleeson, Michael, 10, 70
glucagon, 19–20, 105, 120
glucagon-like peptide 1 (GLP-1) drugs, 127
gluconeogenesis, 9, 31, 103, 114, 138
glucose chews. *See* gummies
glucose performance zone (GPZ), xiv, 43–46, 50–51, 75–94, 150
glucose resets, 91–92
glucose spikes: benefits of reducing magnitude of, 101; complex carbohydrates, 18; data gathering, 33–34, 37; delayed, 84; deliberate, 37, 83–84; "double bump" (biphasic spike), 49; "fake" spikes, 34, 70; glucose gels, 88; and glucose tolerance, 132–133; good spikes, 22, 27, 49, 58, 61; hacks, 29; and the importance of stability, 135; normal glucose responses

after a meal, 79; post-workout, 13, 49, 58, 71–73; priming, 50–51; timing of food intake, 22–29; variability in glucose compared to average, 76–77; worrying glucose responses, 80
glucose tolerance, 35, 98–99, 125, 132–133
GLUT-4 (glucose transporter type 4), 115, 118, 146
glycation, 136
Glycemic Index (GI), 18–22, 124–125, 138–139
glycogen: and adrenaline, 84, 105; cumulative fatigue, 82; depleted stores over a long training block, 59; early morning exercise, 69; and exercise generally, 12–13; exhaustion of supplies, 61; function of, 7–8; and the keto diet, 102–103; "overflow," 82; post-workout, 71; recognizing low, 83; replenishing, 109; and rest, 45; resynthesis, 115, 118; type 1 diabetes, 116, 118; weightlifters, 87
glycogenesis, 8
glycogenolysis, 8–9, 10, 84, 104
glycolysis, 8, 9
Greger, Michael, 137, 140
gummies, 26–27, 58, 66, 100, 106

hacks, 29–32
hard from the gun exercise, 24, 83–84
hard from the start exercise, 41
hemoglobin (HbA1c), vii, 29, 80, 122, 136, 145
high-fructose corn syrup, 18
high-glycemic foods, 18–19, 20, 37–39, 124–125, 131–132, 136, 143
homeostasis, xiii, 25, 27, 34, 61, 75, 79
how to use a CGM, 2–5
hyperglycemia, 7, 11, 12, 114, 115, 116–117
hyperinsulinemia, 12, 114
hyperplasia, 130
hyper-sensitive responders, 90–91, 99–101
hypoglycemia: author's experiences of, vii; and baseline glucose levels, 86; effect on performance, xiii, 6–7, 24, 61, 86; hypoglycemic crashes, 23–25, 39, 61, 62; longer workouts, 58; reactive hypoglycemic crashes, 54, 65–67, 72, 90, 95–97, 105, 113; symptoms, 6–7; type 1 diabetes, 113–114, 115, 118; weightlifters, 68

ideal glucose levels, 67–70
incretin, 134
indigestible carbohydrates, 134
inflammation, xvi, 136, 143
instructions for using a CGM, 2–5
insulin: coordination with glucagon, 19–20; and exercise, 12–13; fats, 132; function of, 9, 11–13; hypoglycemic crashes, 23–24, 25; post-workout, 71; type 1 diabetes, 112, 114–115, 117; type 2 diabetes, 122
insulin resistance: fats, 130–131, 132; vs. insulin sensitivity, 12–13; possible mistaken analyses of, 81, 82; triglycerides, 131; type 2 diabetes, xvi, 111, 122, 125; worrying glucose responses, 80
insulin sensitivity: alcohol, 31; changing, 91–92; cliff, 61; vs. insulin resistance, 12–13; post-workout, 71, 72; reactive hypoglycemic crashes, 66–67; speed of return to baseline, 79; type 2 diabetes, 127
intensity of exercise: fats/proteins, 10, 13, 30; glucose performance zone (GPZ), 45; glycolysis, 8; keto diet, 102, 138; maximal exercise glucose level variability, 84–85; need for carbohydrates for high-intensity, 30, 56; normal effects on glucose, 13; post-workout recovery, 70–71; type 1 diabetes, 114, 118–120; using glycogen, 51, 69; very intense exercise, 56–58; week of hard training scenario, 93–95
interstitial glucose measurement, 1
iron deficiency anemia, 122

Jenkins, David, 138
Jeukendrup, Asker, 10, 53, 70, 118
Julich, Bobby, 24

keto diet, 22, 30, 36, 39, 89, 102–104, 137–138
ketoacidosis. *See* diabetic ketoacidosis (DKA)
ketone esters, 30–31
ketones, 10, 11, 30–31, 112, 117
Khambatta, Cyrus, 122
Kratz, Mario, 131
Krebs Cycle, 10, 11

lab-based blood glucose testing, 35
lactose, 18

lemon/lime juice, 30, 145–146
leucine, 71
Levels app, 5, 6, 77, 123
linoleic acid, 143
lipogenesis, 130, 132
lipolysis, 11, 15
liver, 10, 20, 31, 105. *See also* glycogen
LIVSTEADY®, 55
long training blocks, 58–60
longer workouts, 58, 61, 64–65, 77
low density lipoproteins (LDLs), 135
low-glycemic foods, 18–19, 20, 138–139
lunches, 38, 78

male-female differences, 35, 41, 45, 67
McGregor, Stephen, 7
meal tracking, 5, 33–34
medium responders, 42, 53
medium-glycemic foods, 20
metabolic health, xv, 132–133, 138, 144
Metformin, 126, 145
methionine, 140
monocytes, 130
mood, 14–15, 16, 39, 77, 84
muscle mass, 68, 99
muscle soreness, 70

"naked" carbs, 101, 135
nerves/anxiety, 84, 104, 107, 120
nicotinamide adenine dinucleotide (NADH), 9
non-responders, 87
normal glucose responses after a meal, 79
normal glucose responses during a workout, 62–63
nutritional recovery, 71

obesity, 127, 131
optimal variability, 77
oral glucose tolerance test (OGTT), 133
overeating, 58, 65, 66, 120–122, 127
oxidative phosphorylation (electron transport chain), 10
Ozempic, 127

pancreas, 11, 23–25, 62, 104, 112, 122, 135
parasympathetic nervous system, 15

Performance Manager Chart, 82
"Personal Fat Threshold," 131
pizza and the "double bump," 49
plaque, xvi, 135–136
polysaccharides, 7
post-meal walks, 13–14, 16, 64, 146
post-workout. *See* recovery
preadipocytes, 130
prediabetic stage, 29, 35, 39, 76, 112, 122, 133
pre-event jitters, 104, 107, 120
priming, 26, 50–55, 72, 77, 84, 146
processed food, 139, 140
protein. *See also* keto diet: advanced glycation
    end products (AGEs), 136; benefits of reducing
    magnitude of, 101; and glucose levels, 14, 30;
    Glycemic Index (GI), 22; halting the roller
    coaster, 61, 108; insulin, 11, 80; post-workout,
    71, 72, 73; speed of return to baseline, 81;
    whole foods plant-based diet, 140–141
PUFAs (polyunsaturated fatty acids), 143
pyruvate, 8, 9, 10

RAGE (receptors for advanced glycation end
    products), 136–137
ranges, xiv, 31, 43–45, 56, 75–76, 150–151. *See also*
    glucose performance zone (GPZ)
reactive hypoglycemic crashes, 54, 65–67, 72, 90,
    95–97, 105, 113
Rebelsis, 126
recovery: carbohydrate requirements
    post-workout, 13, 71, 103; eating enough,
    109–110; identifying full recovery, 82;
    protein, 71, 72, 73; recovery phases, 50;
    type 1 diabetes, 115, 118; using a CGM for
    optimal, 71–73
recovery shakes, 13, 58, 70, 71, 72, 110
resistant starches, 141–142
responses, understanding your, 35–43
rest, 45, 82
retrogradation, 134, 141–142
Riddell, Michael, 112, 116, 120
ripeness of food, 21, 138–139
roller coaster, 19, 25–26, 37–39, 58–61, 83–84, 90,
    108, 135
Rothschild, Jeffrey, 50
Ryan, Monique, 70, 71

salad, starting with, 28
saturated fat, 125, 132
second meal effect, 134, 146
seed oils, 28, 125, 132, 143
sensors, 2
sequencing of food intake, 27–28, 141, 150
showering, 34
simple carbohydrates, 18–22, 42–43, 79, 88, 105,
    124–125
Skroce, Kristina, 123
sleep, 1, 14, 34, 36, 75, 115, 118, 123
slow slide, 64–65, 70, 86, 90, 91, 100
slower responders, 42–43, 44, 53, 68, 84
slower-acting carbs, 125. *See also* complex
    carbohydrates
smartphones, 4, 5
snacks, 38
Southerland, Phil, 6, 111, 113
speed of return to baseline, 79, 81
sports drinks, 42, 61, 87–88
sports gel test, 39–41
sports gels. *See* gels
stability, 55–64, 67–70, 76–77, 81–82, 98, 135
starch, 21, 42, 134, 141–142
Stevenson, Aaron, xii, 62–63
stress, 8, 14–15, 27, 33, 119–120. *See also* nerves/
    anxiety
subcutaneous fat, 130–131
sucrose, 42
Supersapiens, xi, 6, 107
super-starches, 88
sympathetic nervous system, 15, 68

temperature changes, 34
testing your glucose response, 35–43
time over and time under, 77–78
timing of food intake, 22–29, 53, 56, 61–62, 77–78
training stress, 70, 82
trend arrows, 118, 119–120
triglycerides, vii, 131, 132, 143, 146
type 1 diabetes, vii, 11–12, 111–128
type 1.5 diabetes, 135
type 2 diabetes: athletic performance, vii,
    122; causes of, 123–125, 130–132; fats, 36;
    medication, 126; reducing risk of, xvi;
    reversing, 124, 127; risk factors, 30

UCAN®, 55, 88, 126
UltraHuman, 3, 6
ultra-processed food, 140, 143

variability in glucose compared to average,
76–77. *See also* stability
vinegar, 28, 30, 145–146
visceral fat, 131

walks after meals, 13–14, 16, 64, 146
week of hard training scenario,
93–95
weight gain, 120–122, 127
weightlifters, 68, 87, 98–99
whole foods plant-based diet, 43, 91, 127, 138,
139–140, 143–144
women, 35, 41, 45, 67

Acknowledgments

....

"... Standing on the shoulders of giants ..."
—Sir Isaac Newton 1676

....

This book is not the work of just one person. It's the work of hundreds, if not thousands, of people sharing their knowledge in books, research papers, articles, videos, conversations, and messages. I am only privileged enough to bring some of that knowledge together into a coherent and systematic way that will help you, the reader, to perform even better as an athlete. I am standing on the shoulders of giants.

First and foremost, Kristina Skroce, MsC, who is the world's expert on CGMs and athletic performance. She basically took me under her wing, read every line of this book, found references, taught me concepts, answered every question, edited every chapter, and was a huge part of making this book great. This book would not have happened without her hard work and dedication in sharing her vast knowledge. I cannot thank her enough.

Dr. Michael Riddell, PhD, is a giant in the diabetes and sports world, having possibly published the greatest number of research papers on the subject. He contributed heavily to Chapter 7 on Diabetes and Athletic Performance, and I am eternally grateful for his epic efforts here. He kept me on the path, focused the chapter, edited it, and added so much to it that he should be considered a co-author of this chapter. Thank you, sir.

My co-author of our book, *Training and Racing with a Power Meter*, Dr. Andrew R. Coggan, PhD, has also helped immensely. He has put up with my innumerable questions, given me excellent answers and references, and inspired me to dig deeper and uncover even more knowledge. I am fortunate to call him a trusted friend.

On my scientific advisory team, Dr. Howard Zisser, PhD, Dr. Gwenael Layec, PhD, Dr. Jamie Whitfield, PhD, Dr. Stephen McGregor, PhD, Dr. Kevin Bernstein, MD, Dr. Diane Reynolds, MD, and Dr. Phillip Kregor, MD, made significant contributions. I am thankful for their willingness to share their knowledge, answer questions, and keep me focused. Each of them contributed in a very meaningful way behind the scenes, which made a tremendous difference.

There are so many athletes that helped with the writing of this book as well. They put up with my crazy requests for their glucose data in various workouts, including hill climbs, sprints on the track, insane early morning sessions in the gym, fasted workouts, high glucose workouts, and epic 12-hour endurance events. I couldn't have done it without each of you, and I am indebted to your hard work and willingness to be a glucose guinea pig! Thank you to Peter Gasperini, Jared Maslan, Aaron Stevenson, Scott Cohen, Rickey Wray Wilson, Michelle Beltran, Gonzalo Olivos, Chris Hill, Lorenzo Elder, Olivia Bradford, Angel Alvarado, Brian Mahoubi, Chris Fay, Michael Stoecker, Stephen Chilmaid, Valerie Hopkins, and Jack Allen.

A special thank you to all the Peaks Coaching Group coaches and staff who helped me gather data, were willing to share their experiences, embarked on wild nutrition theories and tested them, and held down the fort while I went on this adventure. I am blessed with an incredible group of people I call my teammates in this coaching adventure. Thank you to Yvonne Lear, Rickey Wray Wilson, Chris Hill, Dr. David Ertl, PhD, Dr. Stephen McGregor, PhD, Brian Freeze, Paul Ozier, Julie Simmons, Patricia Brant, Keith Nelson, Todd Scheske, Barry Zellmer, and Bryan McKinney.

To Phil Southerland, Phil Bartels, and Bobby Julich, I am deeply thankful for your long-time support, knowledge, advice, and help with everything CGM- and diabetic-related. Without you guys, I wouldn't have gotten on the CGM bus and changed my health for the better, much less have written this book.

A special thanks goes out to my love, Diane, who has inspired me, helped me with gathering glucose data, pushed me to learn new concepts and ideas, supported me in improving my health and nutrition, and put up with all the long hours I put in to write this book.

Finally, thank you to my family for all your support over the years: Susannah Allen, Jack Allen, Thomas Allen, and my biggest fan, my dad, Hunter Allen Jr.

About the Author

Hunter Allen is a world-renowned cycling coach and coauthor of the watershed and bestselling book *Training and Racing with a Power Meter*, which has been translated into 12 languages. He has also coauthored two other books, *Cutting-Edge Cycling* and *Triathlon: Training with Power*.

Widely known as one of the top experts in the world in coaching endurance athletes using power meters, Hunter has been instrumental in developing and spreading the power training principles, traveling to over 20 countries and teaching thousands of cycling coaches and riders. Hunter is a USA Cycling Level 3 coach, was the 2008 BMX technical coach for the Beijing Olympics, and has taught the USA Cycling Power Certification Course since 2005. A former professional cyclist on the Navigators Team, Hunter has been coaching endurance athletes since 1995, and his athletes have achieved more than two thousand victories and numerous national, world championship titles, and Olympic medals.

Ever on the leading edge of tech for athletics, he is a sought-after consultant for many endurance-oriented tech companies and has worked with numerous companies to develop products for the cycling world. Hunter is the codeveloper of TrainingPeaks WKO software; is the cofounder of TrainingPeaks Software; and is the founder and current owner of Peaks Coaching Group.

Hunter holds a BA in economics from Randolph-Macon College and lives in Bedford, Virginia. He has three young adult children, Thomas, Jack, and Susannah. In his spare time, he enjoys driving, racing, tinkering with fast cars and motorcycles, and, of course, cycling around the world!

You can contact Hunter through www.TrainingandCompetingwithaCGM.com or www.PeaksCoachingGroup.com. Follow him on X at @TrainingWithCGM.